Having A Baby
& Other Things
I'm Bad At

Having A Baby & Other Things I'm Bad At

Short stories about living life with infertility

Bailey Henry

Dedication

This book is dedicated to every woman who has known the loss of a child. May you find humor and joy to fill your days, until a child can fill your arms.

You're loved.

And for Aunt Mavis—who told the best stories.

"In three words I can sum up everything I've learned about life: it goes on."

Robert Frost

Contents

Introductions, Disclaimers, and
a Surgeon General's Warning   1

B is for Bent, Not Broken   8

Sitting Shiva   24

Paging Dr. Fabio   41

The Place We Call Redbird   53

And Away We Go   71

A Long December   81

The One Where Everyone Is Pregnant   90

Uncomfortable Comfort and One Less Follower   104

Thanks for Being an F'ing Friend   114

Catch And Release   122

My Mama and Carol King   132

A Table for Two   140

Here I Stand   149

Acknowledgments   154

Preface

A few years ago, I was enjoying a beach vacation with my husband. It was a perfect day on the water. One of those days where you find yourself questioning your real life, and begin going through the ideas of selling all your earthly possessions, quitting your job, and planning for your life to be lived out of a camper on the coast. The sun was warm enough to brown your skin, but not sting it. The water was refreshing enough to cool down, but not shock you. And it wasn't crowded at all. It was one of those perfect days where you couldn't name a care in the world. Well, perfect-ish until I got a sand rash in my bikini area, and then realized that I had dried, crusted chocolate on my chin most of the day. But other than that, it was perfect.

That afternoon was spent drinking mint mojitos and chatting with my husband for the first time in months about anything that wasn't logistic. In between sips of our drinks, good conversation, and dips in the water, I found myself obsessively watching the couple in front of us. Due to my great lip-reading skills, I gathered that they were in town for a wedding, they were from North Carolina, and they were expecting their first child in just a few months. The last piece of information didn't require lip-reading, the woman's perfectly round belly glistened with suntan lotion under the Florida sun. She was petite, and wore a hat that I had been eyeing from the *Cuyana* catalog for months, and she wore it well.

The couple looked happy and well put-together. The husband helped his wife to stand as she walked to the gulf to cool down, and they read books from *his-and-her* iPads. Their love and anxiety was palpable, this would be the last trip that they took before they became parents, and they were discussing how everything they knew was about to change. I'm not a total creeper, their voices carried on the sound of waves crashing, so don't judge me about being nosy.

I wondered what that would finally be like, finding yourself at the end of a pregnancy and not the beginning, reaching the homestretch, and preparing for a new life. I hid my curiosities behind my cheap sunglasses and would peak up every few minutes to watch them, and the hat.

It was a really good hat.

I threw on my cover-up and walked towards the drink stand for a refill, and as I was waiting in line, a voice spoke up from behind me. "Are y'all in town for Anna's wedding, too?" I turned to see the woman I'd been watching stand right behind me. I told her we were just in town for our annual beach getaway, and took the opportunity to compliment the fabulous hat. We made small talk, and I worked up the courage to ask her when she was due. She said early fall, but the baby was measuring bigger, so maybe sooner. I told her congratulations and that I assumed they would be wonderful parents.

"You'll do great!" I said. "I'm sure you both will be good at this." I've no idea why I said it. They were strangers, and there was no way I would've known if they would hit their stride in parenthood or not.

She gave a little shrug and said, "Well, I guess we will find out, right?" Our conversation dug a little deeper as we talked about the anxiety of becoming parents, how hard it is to get pregnant, and the fact that daycare's have a waiting list longer than a gestational period—and that was a whole other issue of worry. She asked me if I had kids and I just said, "No. That has proven difficult for us."

She nodded her head like she understood, but didn't respond. The waiter grabbed my attention and handed me my fresh mojitos. I paid him and began to walk away. "It was nice talking with you," I said over my shoulder. And I again pushed with encouragement that I didn't own.

"Best of luck to you both. I know you will be fine."

"It was nice meeting you, too," she said. Then the beautiful mother-to-be tipped her fabulous hat, and said, "I'm Rachel, and what was your name?"

"I'm Bailey. It's nice to meet you."

1

Introductions, Disclaimers, and a Surgeon General's Warning

When I was in college, I was a smoker. I'm not talking a social smoker who barely inhaled over room temperature beer on *Quarter Pitcher* night. I'm talking: a few over coffee, one before class, a few while we got dressed to go out dancing, two after a big meal, and one before bed. Every day. For about seven years. My roommates and I would sit on our very unstable balcony for hours on end while we lit one off of the other as we solved the world's problems. Those little guys helped me study, and they entertained me on long road trips. They gave me something to do with my hands while I tried to figure out who I wanted to be in this world.

I know.

It's a terrible, disgusting habit that slowly crushes your health and is a dehumidifier for your skin. *But oh, the sweet bliss of that first inhale. Mhmm.* I loved it. Everyone I knew in college smoked. Some of the best conversations and most memorable moments I had in those years were clouded under the smog of *Marlboros, Camel Crushes,* and a few

American Spirits. I've been nicotine free for almost a decade now, but I think back on my tobacco addiction with fondness quite often.

Especially these days. It is currently October 2020. An election year, the year of the pandemic, killer hornets, back-to-back-to-back hurricanes, conspiracy theories, masks, and basically the *anything-that-can-go-wrong-will-go-wrong* year. So yes, I've daydreamed about chain smoking with the windows open to make deciphering Britney Spears' Instagram stories go down a whole lot easier.

But I digress. Why am I telling you about my dirty habit?

Because during my tenure as a chain smoker, when I woke up each morning, a voice inside my head (one of a dozen) would whisper to me gently, *cancerrrr. Lung cancer. Lung cancer. Lung cancer!* And it would remind me of the promise I'd made the day before, that I was going to cut back or quit all together. It was a must. Gone were the days of the glamorous smoker—the *Betty Drapers,* and the *Carrie Bradshaws,* and the *Holly Golightlys* that made the habit look so mysterious and chic. That voice eventually got the best of me, because I did quit. But then, as if she needed something else to do, that same voice that woke me up reminding me of my impending emphysema doom, started singing a new song to me each morning.

The book. Write it. Write it. Write your book, Bailey, she would say to me. For a while I ignored her, just like I did when she tried to convince me to lay down the *Marlboro Menthol Smooths.* Good Lord, do I miss those things. I kept stalling because I thought there could be no worse thing for me to do. Why would I actually follow through on a dream I've had since childhood? And why would I ever write on something that is so gravely personal? If I did that, I would be totally exposed. My heart would be on a page for people to tear or bend or ridicule, and I would feel just about as naked as they come.

But something changed. That voice in my head got louder, and I couldn't focus on much else.

The very idea of moving on with my life and not writing anything felt like I was trying to outrun a train with my foot stuck in the track. I couldn't move forward until I did this. I had been living small, trying not to take up space and disturb others around me, only to realize I was shrinking the idea of my very existence into a box that I didn't build. I needed to stop pushing against the train and, instead, buy a ticket to the woman who I wanted to be. So, I made the very first step and, when the voice called again, I answered.

After I'd experienced two miscarriages, it hit me that this may be my "thing"—my identifier, my battle. I stood in my shower and begged God to please give me another "thing." *Anything but this, God. Anything but infertility.* That voice gently whispered to me, "This is your thing, ok? Just trust. It's going to be alright." When the voice tells you to trust, even if you're terrified, even if it's hard, *just trust.*

Here is the thing about nagging voices in your head: they are usually right. If they are clear and specific and fervent and a driving force for you to make your future days brighter, then they are to be listened to, if not strongly considered. It took me a long time to come to the realization that my drive and desire to share my story is, well, really just for me. I like to think I have a servant heart (servant in the emotional and loving way—not the literal serving way—because also when I was in college, I was a waitress one summer, and I damn near starved after earning no tips because I was so awful) and a welcoming spirit, but that voice has promised me that if I share my story, even just a few of them, then at the very least that will be an investment into the future woman I want to become.

And that is really what our days are all about, right?

Investing in yourself and the people around you to make tomorrow better. If you have a nagging voice in your head that is calling you to enhance your life—to get sober, reconnect with your parents, start a business, start a family, go back to school—answer it. Oblige in the voice just this once. And if that voice is nudging you to lay down a habit that could one day kill you, you should probably do that, too. And as a disclaimer: If the voice is unkind, cruel, or telling you to do harmful things to yourself or anyone else, that is not a voice to be trusted.

Believe me, the very worst version of myself lives in my head if I let her. She is unhealthy and cynical. Crude and harshly judgmental. That particular voice doesn't trust Jesus, and she never laughs. If I let the worst version of me speak up whenever she wants, she tells me not to smile so big because my eyes get squinched, and I look funny. She tells me not to go for my dreams, because I'm sure to fail and nothing good will come of anything I touch. That voice told me not to marry my husband, because surely, I would find a way to mess it up. And that same voice has definitely told me to stop trying to have children, more than once.

The voice of the worst version of yourself will call upon depression and anxiety like old friends who need to catch up over drinks. And that voice is the sort of toxic who can ruin a good day in five seconds flat. I beg you, never listen to that one. Even the ones that say drinking a tea sold by one of the Kardashians will fix all your problems.

They are wrong, they hold no power over you, and they are lying to you.

The positive voice that wakes you up each morning is a gift. For me it is anyway. That good voice is the guiding light that has led me to some of the best decisions I've ever made. Considering how incredibly stubborn and hardheaded I am, the voice begins in my gut and slowly works its way to my brain. No one ever learned a thing from too much wisdom straight out of the gate, right? So, somewhere deep in my core and down in my bones, my soul knows what is best for me before I do. It knew when I was selecting colleges, it knew when I quit my first job, it knew when I looked across a bar and laid eyes on my husband for the first time, and it knew when I opened my computer to start telling my story.

The best piece of advice I've heard is that I'm going to die.

That's a rough one, I know.

One day, the joyful, but monotonous duty of being a human on earth will have ended, and then what? The books you never wrote, the kids you never called, the brother you never forgave, the love you never shared, the songs you never sang, the art you never showed — it will all be gone with you. I know that sounds morbid, but the idea that time is precious and life is a gift and we've only got one shot, well, it really makes you go after life with a vengeance that is gripping. It took years of living small and listening to the negative voice for me to realize that I was wasting precious time.

So here I am, laying out my stories and taking up space. I've been told that I'm intense, and I can make people uncomfortable because I have no filter, and often, no boundaries. I'm okay with that. From the ages of 24-29, I spent the majority of my days comparing myself to others. They looked really happy at their jobs, and I hated mine. Their first homes were bigger than ours. They had more friends than I did. They knew how to draw in their eyebrows better than me. Other women seemed to know exactly who they were, and I was still figuring it out. I played a tiring game of ping-ponging my measure of success and happiness based on other people's Instagram filters. I refuse to do that one more day. And I think you should quit, too.

Breathe deeply, take stock of what your voices are saying to you, and start breaking out of the box you've been told to sit in. Second disclaimer: Do not entirely listen to me, because I'm pretty gullible and believed J.Lo when she said olive oil was the key to her youthful glow.

I'm quite confidant in my brows these days, and I know now that everyone is faking it until they make it. No one knows what they are doing.

I do know for certain that God is more loving and merciful than we acknowledge. I know that sitting outside for an entire afternoon can cure just about anything. I know that the first sip of coffee in the morning is one of life's simple joys. I know that there is no emotion *The Avett Brothers* can't help me feel. I know that a baseball game on a spring afternoon is just about as close to Heaven as it gets. I know that coffee filters make a decent substitute for toilet paper if you ever find yourself in a bind. I know that the best days are still ahead. And I know that once you find good love, love of any kind, you hold on to it until you're dizzy with joy.

And I want you to know that I thank you for being here, and you're loved.

So very loved.

Also, stop smoking and use sunscreen.

Or don't. Do whatever you want.

2

B is for Bent, Not Broken

I remember lying on the exam table. My elevated legs were unshaven and peppered with stubble. My pelvis was pulled forward towards the edge of the table while a quiet technician held a vaginal wand between my legs. I was around seven weeks pregnant and bleeding. She was searching for a heartbeat, a sac, or any sign of life within me. This was the fourth time we'd tried to do this. Fourth loss in a row.

A row.

This wasn't a fluke anymore. It wasn't a string of bad luck like the nurse had told me before. This was my path. My very bleak reality that I couldn't bring myself to face.

My head turned slowly to look at the screen. The image of my uterus projected on the large monitor like I was in a movie theatre. In the short glance, I saw nothing. The black and white grainy image proved to be as empty as I felt—a massive void within me. My gut feeling was validated and with that, we'd come to the end of the road. I broke focus from the screen, and I turned my gaze to my husband. He was holding my hand in an unfamiliar, desperate grasp. In the way you see two men greet each other in the street, clasp hands, and pull each other in with a one-armed hug. Our thumbs overlapped and his fingers seemed to cover my hand entirely.

He held my hand showing he was my teammate, my comrade, my reinforcement; but I hated it.

It was worrisome and foreign. It was how I imaged loved ones hold on to each other during a storm while the roof is ripped from their house. A hurried, desperate grasp in a merciless tornado. He made eye contact with me, and I gave him my knowing look and shook my head. I wanted him to hear the *no* from me. Not from a stranger with her hands between my legs.

But my husband is an eternal optimist and, ever the hopeful, he waited for the confirmation from the technician, which came like an invalid Amazon order. *I'm sorry ma'am. We are all out of healthy pregnancies and babies today. We will let you know when we get another shipment. Would you like an email or a text?*

The sonogram room was warm with recessed lighting and symmetrical art hung under the screen. All design features I usually love, but the single canned light seemed to shine over me and Kyle, illuminating my reactionless face and his glassy eyes. I can remember looking up at the orange glow of that light and thinking to myself, *"Bailey. Life is still good. There will be laughter. There will be wine. There will be dancing, endless discussions, and dirty jokes. There will be travel. There will be joy, damnit."* I was in the middle of that solemn vow just as I felt the sting of the wand leave my body. The technician was silent as she punched in codes and numbers in my chart. I don't think she had looked me in the eye at all. I took her silence as another opportunity to send my husband a message with a cold glare.

Nothing, my love. I'm empty. Again. I'm so sorry.

She told me I could get dressed, and I heaved myself to the bathroom carrying my pants in one hand and clutching my hospital gown closed with the other. My husband waiting by the table, unmoved in a sobering stillness.

He looked beautiful.

I put my underwear and linen shorts back on and knew this wasn't over just yet. I was only spotting, but it was getting heavier; more was to come, the worst was to come. I took a moment to stare at myself in the mirror. My stomach was a bit bloated. My skin was grey. And my eyes—they were brilliant with heartache. My eyelids were so heavy I almost couldn't keep them open. I splashed some water on my face and took a deep breath. I felt so sorry for myself that if I could've given the woman in the mirror a hug, the stench of pity would have rubbed off of me like old perfume.

I came out of the restroom in a fog, and I was handed my chart as my husband stood behind me. The technician made eye contact with me for the first time and said, "Okay, no baby for today. But it's time for you to be strong, little missy! Go upstairs and wait for your nurse to come get you to discuss what comes next. Remember! It's time to be strong."

Are you kidding me? I wanted to scream, "Shut up, bitch. You have no idea how strong I've had to be!" Was that the best she could do? Her eye contact was short lived, and I could tell she didn't believe in her own words.

It's time to be strong.

Her words vibrated over me, and my rage grew. My *strength* wasn't the issue. It was reminding myself to breathe and not to collapse in public that was the challenge. The more suiting advice she could've given me would've been, *"This disaster is not your fault. You're totally allowed to lose your shit. It will be more satisfying if you break things at home and not in public. May I recommend cheap glassware from Wal-Mart. It shatters well. So do lightbulbs and chalk. Oh, and throwing ice cubes at a wooden fence should scratch your itch of rage."*

We waited in a crowded seating area. Women on all sides of me were swollen and glowing while life blossomed within them. Some smiled at me, some didn't. A few gave a humble nod; they had been in my shoes before. I suppose it was my tear-stained face and my husband's pale complexion that gave us away. They should really have separate waiting areas for situations like that. Situations like ours. The pregnant teenagers were oblivious. Their mothers watching me with just as much confusion as I, too, looked on their mere children having children. And there I sat. The adult with a husband, a mortgage, a dog, an IRA, and an Amazon Wishlist, who was currently squeezing my thighs together uncomfortably tight to hold in a blood clot until I could make it to the toilet again. For the fourth time.

The nurse called my name. My husband helped me stand, and we followed her to a room I hadn't been in before. No examination today. No more labs. No more ultrasounds. This was a room for discussion. The art was different in this room. No sign of maternal sketches or pink newborns in here. How kind of them to leave the stale mallard duck paintings for the miscarriage-talk room. There was a golden *B* hanging above the door. "B is for bent, not broken," I said. Not sure where that came from, I put my head down in a middle school embarrassment from sounding like a character on *Sesame Street*. My husband looked up at me and flatly told me it was for the room. "This is exam room B," he said. As we waited for the doctor, I launched into my to-do list of things to finish for the week. I told my husband I was finally going to take the plunge and get Botox. Why not, right? No pregnancy, no baby, may as well eat sushi, drink wine, and beat the cruel hands of time at its own game.

I mentioned that my last two miscarriages lasted about a week or so, so we could still take our vacation in September. His eyes met mine and he shook his head slightly. He reminded me that we hadn't talked to the doctor yet, there could still be hope. Maybe she knew something the tech didn't? Bless his heart. I didn't know if I wanted to kill him or hug him. I'd been telling him since three o'clock that morning when I woke up with blood and stabbing back cramps that it was over. I knew.

Some women know what it feels like to have life pass through them. Some women know what it's like to breathe deeply and feel the heartbeat of a child flutter from their insides. And some know when the flutter stops. I woke him up that morning when I was crying on the toilet. I reminded him again when he was in the shower. I sobbed on the phone with him after he left for work and asked, "Why does this keep happening to me?" The fluttering inside me had stopped. I knew that. Why wouldn't anyone listen to me?

And I reminded him of the tech, the empty screen, her flat encouragement for me to be strong.

Bitch.

Before he could answer, before tears hit my cheek, the
doctor came into the room.

• • •

Seventeen months earlier, I found myself at a friend's baby
shower. While I was getting dressed, Kyle came into the
bathroom and asked me if I was sure about going. "I have to
go," I told him. We had been friends since high school, I
read a bible verse at her wedding, this was her first child—
my attendance felt mandatory. Plus, I'd already shared our
loss on social media. Friends and family knew that we had
suffered a miscarriage in October. A common loss. One in
four women miscarry, and it was especially common in first
time pregnancies. *Blah Blah Blah.*

The comments and likes rolled in like lovebug season in
south Mississippi. I was swarmed with messages until I felt
suffocated. *Prayers for y'all. Love you guys!* And my least
favorite: *You're so brave for sharing. Thank you (kiss
emoji).* I didn't want the attention. I didn't want to be
smothered with sympathy; I hate sympathy. Sympathy is too
close to pity.

My arrogant pride tells me that I'm not one to be pitied. But
I suppose it's none of my business if someone finds me
pitiful.

I didn't want to share our deepest hurt at all, but I just
wanted people to stop asking when we would have kids. I
wanted people to realize their small talk was like taking a
bullet to women like me. I needed women who had gone on
to become mothers to remember what a delicate time it is for
a woman, for a couple, and to remember that she was a
complete person herself, before she was a mother. I am a
complete person, a whole woman, even without children.

I wanted the questions to either stop entirely or be prefaced with something more affable than "Have you thrown out the condoms yet?" Or "When will you plummet yourselves into a sleepless life and crippling debt all for the sake of parenthood?"

Oh, or my absolute least favorite, "Trying is the fun part!"

Please, shut up.

I had marketed myself as strong. I was strong. I am strong. And this common, but hurtful loss would not stop me from being social or supportive of my friends. Not if I had anything to say about it. So, I went, and I smiled. I handed over a gift that2 I couldn't bring myself to buy, instead making my husband go into *Babies-R-Us* alone. He picked the most boring thing off the registry and came out five minutes later.

I watched as my friend beamed in the center of the room. She looked so beautiful. And I kept reminding myself every few minutes that one day, my ship would come in, too. I observed the other women who were mothers themselves giving advice. Some of it sounded solid, some of it sounded like bullshit, but who was I to decide? I could feel my face growing red as she came closer to opening my gift. I knew I should've just faced the baby store and picked something cute. My gift wasn't even wrapped cute. I felt like I was back in high school where everything was a competition. Who brought the best gift? Who had the best wrapping? The best card? The best old wives' tale? The best advice?

My gift was generic and boring. The wrapping was loose and careless. Had I even signed the card? I couldn't remember. And as for advice, well, I had nothing.

I couldn't compete. It was the first time in a long time that I felt like I had no seat at a table. No reason to belong with a crowd of women. And my crushed spirit told me they could see right through me, the barren friend making small talk to hide her shame of empty arms.

As my face continued to flush with heat, I slowly started to step back. And back and back and back some more.

My body was making me take an exit ramp before my mind could keep up. I prepared to apologize to whomever I'd just bumped in to and turned only to see the kitchen wall.

I had gone as far back as I could from the group of women who were bonding over motherhood. Without being able to take any more steps, I felt my shoulders fold into my chest. I was trying to take up as little space as I possibly could. Was it socially acceptable to get in the fetal position on the kitchen floor of a stranger's home? If only I could disappear.

I wondered if I could I sneak out the front door unnoticed. I snickered under my breath deciding that I would tell my husband he was right. How rare I like to say that to anyone, but I would anoint him with the honor of being wise and forthright about my coming here. He was the only person who I felt truly knew me during all of this. His cloudy blue eyes would look at me and he'd say, "You have nothing to prove, and she will understand. You're punishing yourself by going. Please don't do this to yourself." And then I would feel the low hum of his voice give me permission to crumble behind the closed doors of our bedroom.

But I'm a woman, my love! Punishing ourselves is what we do. Endless diets, mom guilt, our inner critics, *Spanx*, overachieving only to tell ourselves we are underachieving, waxing, plucking, injecting, competing, self-deprecating, judging others so we can save time on judging ourselves, and the list goes on. Even the best of our species who would like to think she is above it all, suffers quietly with the pressure she puts on herself. Of course, I went to her baby shower. Of course, I made myself sick on the way there. Of course, I held in my still swollen stomach and pretended not to notice when people stared a second too long, wondering if I was pregnant.

I had a bet to win with myself. And when it's me against me, I have to win.

I was snapped back into the present when my friend looked up and said, "Thank you, Billy!" The nickname she gave me in high school. I saw her brow furrow when she realized I was in the complete opposite room from the actual shower. By then I was as blushed as a child who'd been scolded.

I bashfully played dumb like I'd wandered towards the baby quiches and Presbyterian punch for a refill. As I walked back towards the circle of women to find my place on the sofa, I was overcome with the sense that it would be a very, very long time before I would have a baby shower of my own, and I knew in my bones that I would have to walk through hell to get there.

• • •

When my doctor opened the door, I was taken aback by her sympathy. I know she sees this all the time, but she was the first medical professional who'd actually told me she was sorry that I was going through this. Her tender touch on my shoulder was what tore me that day. The kindness of strangers will undo me every time. From then on, it felt like we were on a launch pad.

Three...two...one...run.

Surgery would be in the morning, don't eat anything after six, three to seven days for physical recovery, God only knows how long on recovery time for a broken heart. I would need to call in to work, drink lots of fluids, no sex for six weeks, do not try again for at least 12 weeks, they will collect the matter left over in my uterus and send it off for testing to understand why this keeps happening.

"You could do IVF immediately and it would probably help, or there is a genetic specialist who can help you, too. We can do genetic testing, hormone testing or hormone therapy, if needed. You have a textbook vagina and a perfect uterus, so our exploration of issues should be fairly easy." My doctor listed off popular reproductive aids and complimented my lady bits as I started to see spots.

Everything felt sterile, including me. The sound of the tissue paper on the exam table, the smell of rubbing alcohol, the not so smooth touch of latex gloves. Nothing felt personal, but everything felt invasive. I wanted to ask my doctor so much more. How will the world know how to help me when I've lost something no one can see? How do I explain to my friends that I'm heartbroken over something I didn't know I wanted so badly? How do I go to the grocery store and see women with their children? How do I not hate myself and blame my husband? I was in love. Where does this love go?

There are things you learn about your own body when you walk through infertility, or any health journey, that maybe the average person doesn't know. I, for one, have a very low sitting cervix, I don't mind the sight of other people's blood (it's my own blood that makes me woozy), and I've learned

that I have an incredibly high tolerance for pain. I also now
know that I have unusually thick skin and child size veins,
which makes my labs and blood work take hours.

I've learned that science can only take us so far with
anatomy, before a belief in the divine takes over. I remember
learning these lessons in a fever pitch. During my first
miscarriage, I was largely in shock. I was shocked to be
pregnant in the first place, we hadn't tried, but we weren't
preventing either. So, when I found myself pregnant only
four months after stopping birth control, I was in a shear
panic.

I was really surprised at myself that I wasn't excited. The
moment the stick turned pink, I could see my life flash
before my eyes. Vacations with Kyle, building our dream
home, all the things we hadn't accomplished yet sped by me
in a hurried laughter. I was left nauseous and defeated. It
took me about two days to settle into the idea of being a
mother. And once the idea was nestled down in my bones, I
realized I would've laid down my life for that child—what a
thought. They were no bigger than a grain of rice, but I
would've chased heaven and earth for them. And just as I
fell madly in love with someone I would never meet, I
doubled over in pain as my body rejected it all.

Never having gone through that before and figuring it was a
bit dangerous to my health as well, Kyle drove me to the
emergency room. It was a Saturday afternoon and
unseasonably warm for October. There was nothing they
could do, so they sent me home to rest and pass it naturally.
But not before serving us with an emergency bill that rang in
right around one thousand dollars.

We were there for 64 minutes.

When I was nearing the end of my loss, I felt an urge to push. I was in the bathtub when a full force labor pain shot through my lower abdomen. I stood up to let nature take its course. I pushed, cried, and braced myself for what I knew I had to do. I fell to the floor and turned to look down to see a perfect embryo sitting on a clot of blood that was the size of a baseball. I knew of nothing else to do but scoop it up and inspect it up close. To see if I could find a heart that wasn't beating. A set of eyes. A resemblance of myself or Kyle. I saw none of those things. I held the perfect form in my hands for as long as I could. I thought about calling Kyle in to look, but a lot of things stopped me from that. I've been told that men don't become fathers until the day their child is born. But women, we become mothers the moment we find out we are pregnant. I had been a mother for a brief moment in time, and I would never forgive myself for not enjoying it from the very start.

I left the doctor's office with a pile of paperwork, a scheduled surgery, and something called *the death stare* that my husband had come to fear.

The death stare is when my eyes glaze over and I zone out for about a week. I don't eat, speak, bathe, or smile. I just check out of life for a while and let my anger and heartache percolate in my chest.

When life utterly shatters you, the checking-out for a few days could be what saves you. It's the staying positive, keep moving, and ignore your feelings mentality that I firmly believe makes us crumble beneath the weight of our expectations. The placing of bets with yourself, the games you play with your own strength and mental health—the games you think you win and never actually do. Life is so reckless with her joy and ecstasy, grief and illness. The

giving and taking of loved ones, victories, securities, and
pride.

Life, in her sheer majestic beauty will absolutely render you
breathless in her blessings, and in her cruelty. The happy
medium, the safe place of surviving, is to sit in the silence of
your own destruction, and watch empathy come to you from
the most unexpected places.

While the death stare is alive and well in our home,
somehow my typically teenage like, helpless husband
becomes *Mrs. Doubtfire*. He can assume my needs before I
can. The dirty dishes he usually never sees somehow
become clean, the dry cleaning is picked up, candles are lit
without me asking, and dinner is made by six. He can make
phone calls and keep the world at bay for me while I fall
apart. God bless him.

Here is the thing about pregnancy loss, or really any loss for
that matter that no one likes to admit: Unless you've been
through it, you just won't get it. Our society has created this
realm of "woke empathy" that is grossly selfish. You can be
an empathetic person and not have all the answers. You can
still sit in the hurt of others and not have the fix-it formula to
spoon feed them. We need to be more comfortable sitting in
each other's hurt and stop waiting for vacancy in the
conversation to tell our own sob story. One upping someone
in grief with a tale of your own, isn't empathy at all.

When you announce that you're naturally pregnant, you're
met with a gambit of lovely and tear-filled reactions. People
buy you blankets and diapers. They purchase the unborn
their first bible or baseball bat. Grandparents start a college
fund before you're in your third trimester. But when you
lose that pregnancy, I was surprised to discover not much is
offered at all.

You're met with a look of sympathy that once again feels like pity. People will change the subject or ask questions in a barely coherent whisper, if they can muster the question at all. Eye contact becomes minimal and your closest friends disappear.

For the same reason you don't make eye contact with the homeless guy on the corner, for the same reason you don't offer to say anything to your friend whose husband just left them, for the same reason you avoid discussions on race or gender equality, it's because *you* are the uncomfortable one.

Not them.

They have to live with their homelessness, their addiction, their shortcomings, their handicaps, their singleness, their infertility.

We live in it. Day in. Day out. We are in it, floating through the what-ifs and worst-case scenarios. We make our beds in the *how did I get here* and the *I can't believe this is happening to me*.

So the next time you want to avoid eye contact with your friend at dinner who is struggling through trauma, addiction, IVF, divorce, coming out, rehab, eating disorders, financial woes, getting dumped, getting fired, being forgotten, or anything else life can hurl at you, look them in the eye and ask them how their soul is holding up. Sit through the thick of their hurt with them. Be there and listen. Don't offer vague advice or flat encouragement, it's been offered before. Be prepared to hear the hurt and triumphs. Settle in for a discussion. Don't fret over hurting their feelings or making them upset. They are comfortably nestled in the hazard zone for the long haul.

The only one who will squirm in their seat, is you.

If you've never felt life literally pass through you, you won't understand this particular type of ache. And that's okay. Grief is so incredibly personal to each of her victims. People will find it copacetic to say the most offensive things cloaked in encouragement, friends of friends will think it's okay to recommend *Kama Sutra* sex positions because they think that is solid advice for fertility, or the worst is when your closest loved ones run from you and hide entirely while you struggle to breathe. But the *death stare*, the falling apart, the sitting in a cold shower for an hour and half, and the glass breaking, and the screaming under water is really what grit is made of.

If we allow ourselves time to break the shit, fall to pieces and not speak until we have something to say, I think that is where we find out who we are. It may sound manic, but when you break anything around you—anything you can get your hands on—and you shatter it down to dust, that is all in an effort to keep yourself from falling apart. And then, only when you're ready, slowly stand up and begin again.

But as anticipated, after you've swept up shattered glass and surveyed the area for damage, you're still helplessly broken. Just like the blue bowl you've hurled towards your kitchen floor. What I wouldn't give to feel the weight of a child on my chest. But I keep that dream of my heart at arm's length in fear that I will not live up to the task.
Like the soldier who steadies his weapon to take aim at the enemy, but whispers to himself not yet. Not yet.

Not yet.

There are no substitutes, no place holders for parenthood.
There are so many space fillers for pleasure or greed or love
and lust to be found in this life. But motherhood—there is
nothing that can imitate that. Nothing can fill that void if the
desire exists within you. This lonely walk is isolating in
itself of heartbreak and embarrassment. But the secret I hold
of coveting those who are parents is deeply guarded by the
safety net of my excuses. *We aren't ready to try again. One
more vacation and then we will. A few thousand more in
savings and then we can go for it.*

I'm dancing recklessly on the tight rope between freedom
and forever. Between falling madly in love with the hope
and idea of a child, and the falling face first failure of
infertility and rejection.

But the truth is, no matter how badly I crave the touch of a
child's hand in mine, I keep looking out on the horizon
waiting to believe enough in myself to say, I am ready.

3

Sitting Shiva

I wish there was a word for what my family did that week. I've searched dictionaries, scriptures, and explained the emotion of events to friends and family. I've scoured the internet to no avail for the word that I thought escaped me, but I don't think it exists. The Jewish faith has the tradition of *Shiva*. Shiva meaning seven and the act of *sitting Shiva* is the weeklong mourning period after a loved one dies where they gather, practice deep prayer, and honor the loved one who left them. While I'm not Jewish, I've always had great admiration for the Jewish community. They are devout in practice, loyal to their faith and community, and certainly know a thing or two about oppression and hard times. I've been searching for my Shiva.

The month before my grandfather died, we all rallied in his home for six days. This wasn't a planned trip, but rather an unexpected spring break that happened in April of 2018. He wasn't dead yet, but after being placed on hospice we could only assume as he would say, "We are in the bottom of the ninth." A few weeks earlier, a nurse came into his hospital room and told him he would be going home as a hospice patient. He responded, "So that means I'm dying." The nurse

tried to ease his worries by saying it just meant he needed
extra attention and many patients have gone on to live life
after hospice. Not convinced, he unclasped his long fingers
and gently shrugged. I believe by then he had made peace
with this life. He held no regrets, and it was very much in his
character to settle on an idea like dying, and not waste any
time.

We didn't do much that week but sit and watch. We catered
to his every need, played music, and put fresh flowers in his
bedroom. We made him comfortable and watched him
breathe. There was a melody of heart monitors and alarms to
remind us to give medicine or check blood pressure. We
watched the sun set over the lake they had lived on for the
last twenty-five years, and we observed our sacred tradition
of cocktail hour. We paid homage to a life that was slipping
through our fingers. That week, while entrenched in beauty
and a peaceful stillness that only comes with death, it was
also fascinating with wonders of the human body,
spirituality, and terror. When the end-of-life phase begins,
fingertips and toes turn purple, and the person approaching
death will pick at their clothing in confusion and have a
fluctuating appetite. Caregivers are on edge and suddenly
have a hard time discerning snores from watery gasps of air.
There is a turbulence about the difference between day and
night, and for an extra layer of emotional fun, they will
begin to have conversations with people who've been dead
for quite some time. You don't know acute spiritual fear
until your grandmother asks, "Who is that behind you?" only
to turn and see no one there.

I opened the back door of their home that entered the
kitchen. The jingle of the loose doorknob, the suction of the
rubber threshold, the clap of the metal blinds on the
window—all the noises of my childhood rushed in with me

as I scanned the house for my family. The familiar smell welcomed me, but I was having a hard time getting my bearings. The house had been different for years, but I hadn't seemed to notice until that very moment. In my mind, my grandparents will always be in that kitchen. Watching pound cake rise in the oven. Laughing or telling stories. Every morning my grandmother would sneak up behind my grandfather while he drank his coffee. He would be reading the paper at the table and she would steal a few kisses from his cheek and giggle at how much she loved him. The sun always seemed to shine in that house, and it had a scent like no other. Somewhere between fresh laundry, pickled okra, gardenias, and *Paul Sebastian* cologne. My coziest memories are known by heart on their small back porch. Coca-Cola's poured over ice with Ritz crackers filled us as we'd shuck corn and snap string beans, while praying for a cool breeze to catch the back of our necks.

The white Formica countertops that were once clean and sparkling were now yellowed with stains of time. The corner of the kitchen island that once housed fresh pound cakes, homemade cookies, and bowls of homegrown tomatoes now held binders of medical records, DNR clauses, last will and testaments, and a first-aid kit that seemed to have run its course. And it was quiet in a way I'd never heard before. The house wasn't silent, but the life and essence that once pulsated from the den to the kitchen was gone.

My eyes darted to the round breakfast table that was once the hub of a bi-weekly poker game that lasted for about sixty years. It was now covered in crumbs and old tissues, fingernail polish stains, and pillboxes that were intimidating. I found my mother at the sink, she was washing dishes in a hurried frenzy, as if a clean plate would soften the blow of losing a parent. I hugged her tightly and she told me that my grandfather was in his bedroom, my grandmother in the

living room, and my cousins were all on their way. I made
my way through the narrow living room and found my aunt
on the phone. She extended her hand to me for a squeeze as I
brushed by. My grandmother sat in the corner with a vacant
face. Her home-health nurse was baby talking to her about
what was on TV. The nurse was a quiet woman with a Cajun
accent who seemed a little too territorial with our kin and
suspicious of our crass humor.

A fine southern woman, my grandmother. I've still not met
too many people with her particular type of southern drawl.
She would use words like *yonder* and *reckon* in everyday
vernacular and you'd not dare think she was being trite. Her
sweet voice was lyrical in its twang, and she had the tiniest
hands I've ever seen. Those hands made the best deserts and
lasagna, were rarely seen without diamonds, could play the
spoons, and could surprisingly hold their own for an arm-
wrestling match with the boys. She wouldn't dare check the
mail without her lips painted pink and couldn't hear the
name Jesus without weeping.

My Mamaw had been fading for years. It started with slight
forgetfulness, then it was confirmed Alzheimer's. The
cruelest way to say a slow goodbye. A creeping breakdown
of habits and motor skills, memories and inside jokes.
Names of your loved ones and your own name slip away.
The same disease that afflicted her sister was now stealing
her away, but when the light went out of her eyes, when she
stopped humming old Methodist hymns, when she withered
away to eighty-eight pounds—we knew her time was
coming. My family just assumed she would go first. She was
older than my grandfather and had lived in a fog of
confusion for well over a decade. When he started to wither,
we wondered if they would leave us in the same season.

I drifted down the hallway to my grandparent's bedroom.
Their house sat on a four-acre lot that overlooked a lake, and
the master bedroom window had the grandest view of all.
When they retired from New Orleans, they were looking for
a quiet country retreat and what they found was a slice of
heaven in south Mississippi. All of our Christmases and
Easters, crawfish seasons and summer slumber parties had
been at this house. We played hide-and-go-seek in the front
yard and climbed oak trees, we took our annual family
picture in the backyard, and we learned to fish off their dock.
My husband and I even exchanged our vows on the shore of
the lake. That house is special, the lake is like a peace-
offering to our souls and regrettably, you never appreciate
such things until they are memories.

Their bedroom was bleak. The king size bed was turned
down, and the once well-decorated space was now a grey
time capsule. Boxes of medicine and ointments, gauze pads
and latex gloves lined the top of the dresser. I looked over at
the bed that could hold five of us at once.

My summer nights as a child would end with my cousins
and me in a dog pile watching *Matlock*, *Murder She Wrote*,
and our all-time favorite—*Walker Texas Ranger*. I blushed
with embarrassment as I came through the door. In my
hospice naivety, I figured my grandfather would be resting
in his own bed, the one he shared with his bride. But there he
was in a hospital bed over by the window. *Sleeping. Stilling.
Dying.*

My mom had called a few weeks earlier. She had been her
parent's primary caregiver for years by then. Cooking their
meals, cleaning their home, bathing her mother and applying
ointments in not so friendly places. But lately her father had
taken a turn downhill and he was picking up speed. I
answered the phone to hear silence only interrupted by slight

whimpers and gulps of air. "He's dying," she cried. My
grandfather. A strapping six foot three, black haired, blue
eyed, Alabama-bred stud was running out of sand in his
hourglass. I thought she was being dramatic, because it
wasn't until that moment that I ever considered he could die.
Bill Massey was one of those people who I just assumed
would live forever.

R. W. Massey grew up dirt poor in the sticks of northern
Alabama on the heels of the Great Depression. He was the
son of a farmer and a home maker, and the second oldest of
six boys. He graduated high school at the age of sixteen and
immediately went to work for the school driving a bus. I get
wild eyed with laughter when I think about a sixteen-year-
old boy driving around thirty children with no seat belts on a
school bus; something that would surely never happen today.
My grandfather was painfully shy as a child, and he recalled
being extraordinarily hungry for the first ten or so years of
his life. His mother was a practical joker who adored pulling
pranks on her boys, and his father committed suicide just
before my grandfather left for the army, from which he
would never recover. He was very wise and a hard worker,
handsome and punctual to a fault. He poured two fingers of
scotch over ice every day at five o'clock and if you paid
close attention under his bushy coal black eyebrows, he had
light blue eyes that twinkled with mischief. And he could
strike a match on the bottom of his shoe.

I tip-toed to his side and balanced myself on the corner of
his bed, taking up as little space as I could. He looked the
same, but so different. He was still so tall, but now so frail. I
looked out the window to see the sun set on the water and
could feel the tears begin to bite.

How did it go by so fast?

Weren't we just here?

I was a kid just a minute ago helping him fish and pick
blueberries.

He stirred in the bed as the smell of medicine and saline
water steamed from his oxygen tank.

His wrinkled eyelids slowly opened and when he saw me, he
grinned. As long as I live, I will never forget that cheeky
grin. I swallowed my tears in an effort not to upset him, but
again in my ignorance about death, I didn't realize he could
hardly see anymore.

Life in her final days is a literal blur.

"Hey you," he croaked.

"Hi Pappaw. I missed you."

He scrunched his eyes and straightened himself. I grabbed
his hand and was totally prepared to sit in silence, breathing
him in and watching the water dance through the window.
Instead, he became more alert and studied me. I just knew
this was it. We were going to have one of those talks. It
would go down as the conversation of my life. My
grandfather, on his death bed. Me, waiting for the last bit of
love and advice to pour from him.

I would one day tell my children about this talk.

He squeezed my hand and stared at me. I steadied my heart.

"Is that necklace real gold?" he asked.

What?

"If it's real the price of gold should be on the up and up by the end of the year. You could sell it and make a profit."

No, not quite dead at all.

By that evening we were all home. With our stocks of food, liquor, adult diapers, and heart monitors, we prepared for the week ahead and braced ourselves for the waves of grief that come before, during, and after loss. We called neighbors and old friends from Louisiana to come visit and say their goodbyes. Hundreds of pictures were scattered over every table in the house, just waiting for their story to be told. The one time my grandfather and his brother had to bury a dead donkey in the summer heat, the times when he had to hitchhike from Indiana to Alabama while he was in the army, and the many images of he and my grandmother together. A love story told over sixty-seven years was reduced to polaroids in a shoe box. It was impossible to look at the pictures of them and not hear their laughter.

Hospice nurses and sitters came in and out of the house over the week. Some were so kind and loving that I didn't want them to leave. I was comforted by their compassion and knowledge of how to care for the elderly. Others were lazy and treated my grandparents as if they were burdens, undeserving of care. One afternoon, my aunt and I went into town to pick up lunch. When we returned, the sitter had all the lights turned off as if to hurry them to sleep and she was watching *Women Who Kill* on the Discovery Channel. I was furious. If my people were so close to death, then I would be damned if the last thing they saw in this life was a dark and empty home and images of some woman named Heather

setting her husband on fire. The job that was clearly not fit
for some, was the calling of love for others.

One evening, early in the week, things came boiling to a
head. It had been a long day, and we all were ready to turn in
for the night. My mom and her sisters had essentially moved
back home with their folks. They would take shifts during
the day and night to check oxygen levels or coax my
grandparents back to sleep, run errands, and monitor
temperatures. They were exhausted. Their lives had been put
on hold to watch their parents break the veil between heaven
and earth. But on this particular evening we were down to a
skeleton crew. Myself, my mother, her sister Debra, and my
cousin Ashley were on duty. That morning one of the
hospice nurses taught me how to use something called a
transfer board. It looks like a large cutting board that you
would find in a kitchen. But it is used to help you move
someone from a chair to a wheelchair, or wheelchair to the
bed. This is a simple four-step process.

You ask the patient to lift one hip, if they can, then you
scooch the transfer board under their bottom. Then, firmly
placing the other side of the board on the destination surface,
the patient can slide down the board safely. This prevents
stressing the patient with falling or an even bigger disaster.
This process sounds simple enough, but the nurse failed to
mention the severity of transferring a big-boned man who
was still well over 6'2. Additionally, she didn't give me the
play-by-play of transferring said man who was attached to a
catheter and drainage bag. I wish I could say we at least
started off on the right foot, but that would be doing a grave
disservice to the truth.

My mother, a woman who considers all directions and rules
as needless suggestions, approached the situation with the
same gusto as she approaches life—*directions are for losers*.

I'm not sure what she was focused on while I was
screaming, "Bag, bag, the pee bag, mother!" But she didn't
hear me until the wheel of my grandfather's motorized chair
was rolling over the drainage bag and the hose popped off,
leaving a sort of irrigation issue on the carpet. It flapped and
fluttered in the same coil that a water hose does on the lawn
when there is too much water pressure.

Okay, we can clean that up later.

Ashley and Debra stood behind my grandfather to balance
him as I wedged the board under his lifted hip. Without the
presence of the hospice professional, the *scooch and slide*
steps were now more like, "Balance, don't drop him! Are
you okay? Are we hurting you? Oh, Pappaw I'm so sorry!"

He was patient and gracious as we struggled through. Beads
of sweat began to glisten on our foreheads as we helped him
push himself down the board and slump from the couch to
the wheelchair, then quickly throw the thing in reverse, and
hightail it to his bedroom. Rolling over his own catheter and
taking out a chunk of the wall in the process. At times, his
movements resembled strength and agility, and other times
he looked like *Weekend at Bernie's*. We may have broken
even in that battle, but we were about to lose the war. We
now had to transfer him from the wheelchair to the hospice
bed, change his clothes, dress his bed, and do all of these
things while leaving the man with some dignity. We tried
with all our might to be tender and respectful. If Ashley
could have gone blind that night, I think that is the route she
would've chosen over seeing our grandfather in the buff.
She playfully straightened the curtains behind the bed and
counted cracks in the ceiling to avoid seeing something that
was sure to haunt her for years to come. Laughter helped.
Laughter always helps.

There is a level of humility that is found in moments like this. All humans will face a time where they may consider themselves too prideful to be bathed by their grandchildren. Or too important to help a loved one go to the bathroom or wash their hair. All egos and arrogance of self-importance were checked at the door. My grandfather never once barked an order to us while we *Lucy and Ethel'd* our way around him. And as for us, the women who took care of him that night, we all considered it an honor to love and care for both he and my grandmother while they excused themselves from this life and prepared to enter the next.

That week continued through laughter and tears, backaches from lifting him, and heartache from realizing my grandmother had not only stopped eating, but speaking, too. We kept the moral up by dancing throughout the house during the day and giving each other frequent hugs and thank-you's.

Thank you for being here, thank you for taking out the trash, thank you for going to the store, thank you for doing what I can't, thank you for all of it.

But at night, when the cicadas fell into harmony with the chirps of a breathing machine, I was overwhelmed with the desperation for more time. I shot out of bed from a deep sleep one night in a heated panic because I realized I was watching my mother and her sisters prepare to live in a world without their parents, and I one day would have to face a world without mine.

The world felt vast, and I was falling with no safety net. It was a feeling of needing to hold on to someone who wasn't there, as if the love I craved had already been consumed, and there was no more to give or receive.

I was breathing but taking in no air.

I'd faced my mother's mortality once before. When I was seven years old, my mother was diagnosed with breast cancer. Her battle with the disease is like a relative in my childhood memories. Like an old aunt who was always around and ended up in a few pictures. Not always in the forefront of my recollections, but never far. When I look back on my childhood there are definitive chapters.

Before or after we moved from New Orleans to Mississippi.

Before, during, or after Mama's chemotherapy.

Before, during, or after her second diagnosis, which came just four years later, and so on.

I didn't know any other kids my age with a mom who had cancer. But then again, my mom didn't know any other healthy thirty-six-year-old women who had to ask their husband to shave their heads on the back porch either.

Not long after my mother found a lump in her breast, she had a lumpectomy. I can vividly remember my father begging her to go ahead and have a double mastectomy straight away. My mom didn't want to lose her breasts, and now that I'm almost the age she was when she was sick—I can't say any of it would be an easy decision.

The evening after her lumpectomy, I walked to my parents' room to say goodnight. Their master suite had a wall dividing the bedroom from the bathroom with an open arch entry connecting the two. As I stood in the doorway of the bedroom, I could look to my left and see my mother. She was lying on her back sobbing and writhing in pain. She cried out, "It hurts. It hurts."

They'd taken a third of her left breast and stapled back what remained. As I stared at her yelping under the sheets, I could also see my father on the right. He was running the sink at full blast to muffle the sounds of his own sobs. A husband on one side of a wall, crumbling at the idea of losing his wife, seeing her in pain and not being able to help her. A wife on the other side, unaware that her spouse is aching for her healing. Both not knowing that their daughter watched from the doorway.

Somehow, I found facing the loss of a parent easier as a child than I did as an adult. Maybe it was the faith of a child against the denial of a grownup. But all I knew that night as I calmed my breathing in the dark hallway, was that if I wasn't promised more time with my family, I would not waste whatever time we had left.

For a long time, my oldest cousin, Jonathan, was a perpetual frat boy. I mean this in the most loving way. He is the most successful *Peter Pan* I've ever known. Between his very successful corporate career and string of broken hearts, (theirs, not his), he has the striking good looks of a Kennedy and the sense of humor of Van Wilder. Not much in this life could bring him to his knees the way Faye Massey could. He was the first grandchild, a pride and joy. There is a picture of my grandmother holding Jonathan at my parents' wedding. She was twirling him around the dance floor as my grandfather watched. Twinkles of contentment in all their eyes.

He towered over her by two feet, and he could make her laugh until she cried.

In the six days that we nested together there were a lot of laughs and triumphs, but many a downfall as well. My grandmother not eating was certainly a downfall. It worried us to no end that her body was starving and frail. One afternoon, Jonathan labored over a shrimp and grits concoction. A good Louisiana boy to his core, he just knew she would eat that classic. He carefully boiled the grits down to a creamy consistency and added just enough butter and seasoning for her 90-year-old taste buds to enjoy, but not be overwhelmed or upsetting to her stomach. The moment came for him to serve her in the living room. He had checked the temperature, the seasoning, the texture. It was perfect. He bent down to put the bowl in front of her and encouraged her to try it. She took one bite and grimaced in disgust, shaking her head. "Well, I'll just go fuck myself," Jonathan chuckled. We all laughed so we would forget to cry. No dice. Another day passed and no food consumed.

With each passing day, time was dense. By that weekend I shared the exhaustion my mother and her sisters had known for months. I don't know how they kept it up. Tending to their parents, taking care of those who took care of you for so long, the shoe now on the other proverbial foot. The saying an interminable goodbye each day for months on end. The commitment, the love, round the clock care—it is selfless and admirable. That Saturday, the weather was idyllic. We opened the doors and windows to let the spring air diffuse the stagnant house. My aunt Denise dressed my grandmother in her pearls and summer hat, and we covered my grandfather's legs in a blanket so he wouldn't get sunburnt. And we all headed down towards the dock. The sky was perfectly clear, and it almost seemed as if my grandmother was making memories, too. One more for the road.

There is a very tangible presence that occurs right before a
hurricane makes landfall.

Not the *calm before the storm* feeling that arrives the day
before, but the quiet stillness and almost airless feeling the
hour before. The deafening quiet that falls under a blanket of
inertia. Between the rays of sunshine and the quiet laughter
of a family on the water, the day felt like that. There was
peace, and there was a finality in the air that was immovable.
In the wee hours of the next morning, my grandfather awoke
in confusion.

Scratch that.

It was only confusing for us and only for a second. He spoke
clear as day in short sentences as if he was on the latter half
of a conversation.

My aunt Denise was there to whisper him back to sleep.

"Everything has stopped," he said.

"What is it, Daddy?"

"Everything. I've got to go. I'm going on a trip soon. To
Heaven, I think? There is no more. Everything has stopped."

Later that day, he hardly opened his eyes, but in his mind, he
began to prepare for this trip he talked about. His big hands
were steady as they ran an invisible comb through his hair
and straightened a tie and suit coat that only he could see.
Unmistakable movements with empty hands. Once he was
dressed, he placed his hands by his side, and he whispered a
very clear *Hallelujah*.

By the next evening, I was back home. My mother called
from my grandfather's side, and he sounded tired but a little
more lucid than he had the night before. When I left them
that Sunday, the house was busy. Nurses and neighbors were
in the kitchen, my cousin David and his wife were packing
up to leave, too. I hugged my grandparents goodbye, only
assuming it would be the last time I embraced them on this
side of Heaven. My grandmother felt like a child in my
arms. Skin on bones and so frail I could have sworn she was
going to break in half.

I didn't get a chance to say the things in the hurry of my
leaving. The final things I needed them to know before they
left us. So when I answered the phone, and I heard him in
the background, I asked my mother to put the phone close to
his ear, so he could hear me one last time. I wasn't going to
assume he knew. I was going to make sure he heard me.

"Hey Pappaw, it's Bailey. Listen, I just needed to tell you
that you've made my life so special. You were the best
grandfather a girl could've asked for, and I hope you know
how much I love you. You and Mamaw are some of the
greatest people I've known, and it's been an honor to be
your granddaughter. I love you so much. I hope I can see
you soon, ok? But just know you've meant the world to me."

"I love you too," he said.

"The pleasure was all mine."

My grandmother slowly rolled her walker up to the side of
his navy-blue casket. Clarity greeted her for the first time in
months, and as confusion left her face for a fleeting second,
she turned to us to ask, "Is that my Bill?" Before her tears
were dry, she had forgotten why she was sad. And for the

next nine months she would forget over and over and over
again that she was a widow.

We all took our private moments to say goodbye to his
vessel.

I squeezed my mother's hand as we looked down on him one
last time. He was so thin that all the bones in his face
seemed huge.

"Mama. They were supposed to bury him with his teeth in, I
don't think they are in."

"They are in. He just got so thin you can hardly tell."

"No, there is no way. Look at his mouth. It's so gaunt."

"Sweetie, no. If his teeth weren't in, his chin would be
touching his nose."

At the graveside, a young serviceman played *Taps* on a
bronze trumpet and it was hauntingly beautiful. Pieces of
dirt and sand gently fell from the mound as two soldiers
folded an American flag in perfect accord in front of us, and
they turned to face my grandmother. She had been mute for
months, starving for weeks, and was blissfully unaware that
her husband was being lowered in to the ground in front of
her. But as the sergeant leaned forward to tell her that her
husband's service was appreciated on behalf of the President
and the United States Army, that frail and broken-hearted
woman used all her strength to stand up, look him in the eye,
and take the flag in her arms.

4

Paging Dr. Fabio

I stared at my fat fingers as I sat quietly in the parlor of my hometown funeral home, waiting for my cousin David to walk through the door. My fingers were still swollen from my third miscarriage that happened the month before my Mamaw died. I was trying to twist my wedding rings loose, but I was becoming increasingly pissed that they were stuck and supremely pissed that I was the type of woman to swell upon conception. David and his very pregnant wife, Chelsey, were coming in from Louisiana for my grandmother's service. Since childhood, I've always felt an odd responsibility to greet David at the door as he arrived. Call it hospitality or good manners, but it comes from a bit of a selfish place. When we were kids, David was the family entertainer. He could do a wicked spot-on impression of Jim Carrey in any role from *Ace Ventura*, *The Mask*, or *Liar, Liar*. He was a quick-witted child who usually managed to get out of trouble because adults can't run fast when they are bent over in hysterics. His presence was always a comfort to me because I knew that after we hugged and said our hellos, laughter was never far away.

Once they arrived, we had a private viewing of my
grandmother before the service began. We opened the doors
for guests to tell us they were sorry for our loss, and I found
it refreshing to not pretend that I was sad for other people. I
would miss her forever, but I was so thankful my sweet
grandmother was no longer suffering. About halfway
through the receiving line, I could see a former teacher of
mine making her way to me. She smiled and gazed at the
adult in front of her who'd replaced the clumsy, third grade
girl she remembered me to be. She gave me a warm hug and
politely asked me how old I was, if I was married, and if I
had children. I introduced her to my husband and told her I
was twenty-nine and holding. I was just about to ask how
she was doing in an effort to skip her last question, but she
held on to it. "And what about kids?" Her face lit up like I
was going to give birth right there in front of her. I smiled
quietly and dusted off my standard answers.

Oh, not yet. Maybe one day.

We are enjoying being married for now.

*We've thought about it and look forward to it when the time
is right.*

Those answers usually cover my truth of wanting to scream,
"I will have a baby when my body can carry one to full term.
Now sit down, Janet."

None of my answers satisfied her, and she wouldn't relent.
"Oh, come on! I know your parents would be beside
themselves. Give them grandbabies while they can still
enjoy them!" Ah, the added responsibility on women to give
our relatives children. I stood in front of her thinking back
on the times I'd told our families we were pregnant and then
hiding behind our phones to tell them through text that we

weren't anymore. My face flushed red with a heat that wasn't familiar. I typically change colors when I'm under pressure, but I could even feel my eyes puffing with fever. I fake laughed at her persistence and finally stumbled out words that sounded choppy, like my mouth had bad cell service. "I... we...we...miscar...we have trouble with that."

Hoping she would share some of the embarrassment I was currently suffering, she only launched into a story about a friend of a friend who adopted from China. I was stuck with no way out. I felt like the third grader she remembered and wanted to give myself a timeout. Maybe if I stuck my nose in the corner of the room that would satisfy her. I was weighing my options of pretending to faint or considering how she would handle an upper cut to the chin, when laughter erupted from behind us.

The whole parlor fell silent as we all turned to see David entertaining a circle of visitors on the other side of the room. When I turned back around to face my teacher turned interrogator, she was gone. I was saved by David's comedic timing once again.

Over the next few days, I would be suddenly struck with waves of the same fever and heated cheeks. The fever would start almost every afternoon like clockwork and along with the rising temperature, my face would be as red as a slapped ass. I found myself putting ice cubes on my cheeks to find relief from the heat. My eyes would be swollen and tired, and I would lose all energy. I wrote it off as a head cold, exhaustion, or a new way my body had found to manifest depression. I lived with a daily fever for over two weeks when finally, I came to my wits end and went to the doctor. I didn't know how else to explain my symptoms other than being tired and having a random fever. I answered all of the nurse's questions about medication and medical history and was unsettled at her shortage of possible diagnoses. "It doesn't sound like the flu? And you're sure you don't have any other symptoms other than fever and a hot face?"

She gave me a cup for a urine sample and showed me to the restroom. I closed the door behind myself and was surprised to see nothing but a toilet and a stand-alone sink. There was no counter or chair to put my jacket and purse on. No diaper changing table for moms-on-the-go. Not even a coat hook on the door. I'm a firm believer in never putting your belongings on a public floor, so I stood there staring at the toilet mapping out my course of action.

I guess it's time to share a little fact about me. I'm a spoiled pee-er. I need a sink and a cute table, or a countertop with candles and soap dishes. I need a well-lit mirror and paper towels fully stocked. We've all got our base demands, and those are mine. One hunting season a few years back, Kyle thought it would be fun to take me on a day long hunt. When he told me that I would have to go to the bathroom outside while holding on to a pine tree and manage not to get stung or poked with anything, well, let's just say he never let me wear his coveralls again.

A lightbulb went off, and I patted myself on the back with genius. I would take the handles of my large tote and hang it around my neck like an Olympic medal, and it would rest in my lap.

Check.

Then I would keep my coat on and take its end corners up and hold them in my left arm, while I peed into the cup I was holding in my right hand.

Check, Check.

I popped the lid off the urine container and almost placed it on the sink, but thought better of it. Sinks are dirty. But where would I place the lid while I complete my obstacle course of peeing? My mouth, obviously. I held the lid between my teeth and carefully placed my purse handles over my neck and clutched my coat in my left hand and balanced the cup in my right.

Here goes nothing.

I suppose I had one too many cups of coffee that morning, because heavens to Betsy if my tee-tee didn't come out at twenty miles an hour, knocking the cup out of my hand and into the toilet.

Shhhhhhiiiiiiiitttttt.

I leaned to the right as my arm received a golden shower and I fished for the cup that was now mostly filled with toilet water. I dumped it out and prayed my test wouldn't come back to say I have chlorine poisoning. My purse was swaying around my neck giving me a sort of rub burn and when I looked down at the lid that had fallen from my bite when I started laughing at myself, I thought, "All this for a stupid fever." I carefully put myself back together, thoroughly washed my hands, and handed the nurse my sample that was no more than a droplet.

The family physician came in the exam room and told me that my sample was fine (that was a miracle), blood work was clear, and they had no reason to believe I was contagious. The nurse had checked my temperature earlier and of course, I was at 98.6. The doctor was recommending drinking more water and lots of rest when I could feel my color change. His head tilted and he asked me if I felt fevered right then. I did. He took my temperature again and 100.7 flashed on the thermometer. "So, each time your fever spikes, your face flushes and gets red at the same time?" Yes! I was so excited he was able to witness this in live action, maybe we could finally get somewhere.

"My dear, I believe you have parvo." *Parvo?*

"Like, what puppies get?"

I learned that day that the parvo virus shows up mainly in children and the elderly. Commonly known as *fifth disease*, it can leave you with a rashed face and pesky fever for weeks, it can also be harmful to pregnancies. I received a steroid shot and antibiotics and went home retracing my steps of where I could've gotten such a virus. I drove home in silence considering how long I may have had it and if this is the reason I miscarried just five weeks earlier.

We always look for something to blame. We hold our burdens in our tote bags waiting for the right moment when we can hand them off to someone or something else. Anything to get the weight off of our own shoulders. The biggest obstacle in looking where to place our blame, is just finding a suitable scapegoat at all. How are we to ever make it through life just accepting the nothingness of fate or just accepting the cards we are dealt? We spend hours of days we aren't promised looking for answers that may not exist. There is nothing to blame, except usually, we blame ourselves. When I got home, I stood in my bathroom mirror and couldn't even recognize myself. My face was still beet red, my hair dry and frizzy, and I had officially gained so much weight that I got winded just getting dressed. At

twenty-nine years old my health, which I'd taken for
granted, was now turning its back on me.

Cruel words of blame and fault were used as weapons, and I
started beating myself to a pulp.

*No wonder you can't carry a child, look at you. You can't do
anything right.*

*How can you even go anywhere? You're embarrassing your
husband.*

You don't even look like the same person you once were.

People are thinking you've let yourself go.

You're pathetic.

You are really bad at peeing.

I'd become familiar with the routine of camouflaging myself
from the world. Wear baggy clothes, preferably black or
grey, apply extra makeup, don't speak unless spoken to, if
you pose for a picture make sure you are hiding behind
someone or something, do as much of your job as you can
via email and phone calls. I'd stopped checking in on friends
and family, because a voice in my head told me they didn't
want to hear from me. In many ways, I'd stopped living.

I was arriving at the place I'd always feared I would stay, the
hub of passivity. I was passive—a secondary co-star to the
leading lady. But if I wasn't leading my life, who was? I was
beginning to accept commonality for my life, and I knew
that it felt wrong. My life, all lives, are made for so much
more than playing second fiddle to who you could be. Just

before I began to fully hate myself, the phone rang. My first two miscarriages were pretty much ignored by my doctor. "They are so common. I usually don't do any testing until you've had three or four."

Three or four?

Have you ever had just one? Because I can assure you, they wreak enough emotional havoc on a woman that you would want a full body scan after just one. That OBGYN even prescribed a progesterone vaginal suppository for my second pregnancy that was coated in peanut oil. The only problem is that I'm deathly allergic to peanut oil. I guess the fine print of my patient chart wasn't worth reading. The last phone call I had with her nurse was a conversation in which I was sobbing, and she was laughing.

"Yes, I have an appointment on Monday, but I miscarried over the weekend. Can I still keep my appointment and y'all just check me out to see if I need a D&C or if there is anything going on down there?"

The nurse snickered and produced a nasally laugh as she coldly said, "Umm, how far along were you? Oh, just six weeks." *chuckles again* "No, we don't do that. You're fine. We will see you for your annual checkup in April."

But I wasn't fine.

I was furious and devastated. I was abusing my body with food and alcohol, and I constantly felt like shit. I had a persistent fever, I couldn't sleep, and my hair was the texture of pine straw. I was not fine. I answered the phone and remembered that I had called a new doctor for an appointment and her nurse was calling to confirm. This was it.

I was getting somewhere. I was finally going to be listened to, and have tests run, and actually learn what my blood type was, and all the things. They had a cancellation that day, and it was just my luck that I was next on the cancellation list and had a free afternoon.

Answers were just around the corner.

I sat down in the small waiting room and pulled out my phone to Facebook stalk my potential new doctor. She went to medical school in California, she was a young mom who was part of *La Leche* forums, she advocated for women, and she had a filter on her profile picture that boasted a marijuana leaf in support of passing medical marijuana bills. She gave the social media appearance that she was chill, but aggressive towards fighting for, and listening to, women.

I couldn't wait to meet her.

She burst into the room with fresh energy and wild curly hair. I noticed a tall young kid behind her who looked like he had just come in from surfing a gnarly wave, dude. His long blonde ponytail laid over his chiseled shoulder, and I was jealous of his sharp bone structure and golden tan. She introduced herself and turned to Fabio behind her and said he was a medical student. "Would you mind if he sat in on our consultation?"

"No, not at all," I told her. I was grateful to have two sets of ears listening, and maybe between the three of us, we could figure out what was going on. She began to review my medical forms and asked a ton of questions. My mother's history with cancer, my miscarriages, family history of diabetes, and so on. After going through my grandfather's

history with skin cancer and just before I started on my
current list of symptoms, she stopped me.

"Can I be perfectly honest with you?"

Dear God, yes. Please be honest with me. I was bracing
myself for her to send me to a specialist or tell me that she
thought I would never carry a child to full term, I just
wanted something to stand on. She grabbed my hand in hers
and held a long dramatic pause. Ahh, it's happening.
One way or another I'm getting answers, baby.

"I think you're being a little neurotic, and I think you need to
just chill. You've been through a lot and I suggest you have
a glass of wine and just let your body heal." Dr. Fabio
nodded in agreement behind her. *Neurotic? Wine? Chill?*
But I hadn't even gotten to the part where I was going to tell
her I was using wine as a band-aid to heal from trauma. I
was chilling so much that I felt like I wasn't living. How was
this supposed to be helpful? She didn't have a cold,
snickering laugh like the nurse from the other doctor's
office, but this hurt just the same. And I had no one around
me to tell me that she was wrong.

She was a doctor. A professional. She went to medical
school, I didn't. She had delivered babies in the Congo, I
hadn't. I resigned to the fact that she knew best, and I
didn't—even when it came to my own body. I couldn't
diagnose myself with parvo, I couldn't give myself a scan of
my uterus, and now a doctor who came highly recommended
was telling me to just chill.

I was humiliated. I gathered my things, shook her hand, and
told her it was nice to meet her. If I'd known then what I
know now, I would've stood up for myself. Or at the very
least, told Dr. Fabio that women who prioritize their health

are not neurotic. I can only hope he didn't go back to med-school and tell his friends about the great bedside manner he was learning. I searched for a silver lining and was relieved that I didn't have to pee in another cup that day. I felt foolish and unconvinced. I'd never had a reason to not believe a doctor and was unfamiliar with the feeling of trusting myself over a medical degree.

At another point of desperation, I called my real estate agent, Cate. In conversations had over selling our first home, she relayed to me that she had seven losses herself. This was before my own experience, and so I didn't know how to connect with her over such a thing. But I was so grateful for her that day.

"Bailey, are you kidding me? No, you're not neurotic. You're sad and you want answers. I know loss is common, but usually not consecutive and even so, if you feel like something is off with the body that you've lived in everyday for twenty-nine years, then something is off. Find a doctor who will listen to you."

But wasn't I supposed to listen to them? I'd never thought of such a concept. I wanted a doctor's opinion, but I also needed a doctor to hear me when I said I felt like I was drowning and something wasn't right.

Turns out, Cate was right. When you live inside your own body and feel like something is off, something is usually off. I found a doctor who finally ran plenty of bloodwork on me and, together, we started to figure some things out. This process took over a year.

First off, my thyroid was in major distress. And to my
surprise, your thyroid is a pretty big deal when it comes to
fertility.

That explained the dry hair, ruddy skin, mood swings, and
weight gain. I have a blood clotting disorder that affects
pregnancies, and as it turns out, I do not have a tilted uterus.
We were gaining ground and finding answers. I was being
heard and she even suggested that I put myself in therapy to
slowly claw my way out of the hole that I had buried myself
in. I slowly found my voice and had to remind myself to not
say, "I'm sorry, I just have a few more questions." I
shouldn't be sorry for inquiring about my own body. And
neither should anyone else.

Apologies and anatomy should not collide into each other on
the road to recovery. Women should be confident enough in
their autonomy to ask whatever they want, whenever they
want, however they want.

How will the universe ever know what you need, if you
never ask for it? *Ask for it.* And take it from me, if you ever
find yourself needing to provide a urine sample in a
restroom with just a toilet, ask if they can hold your purse
behind the desk.

5

The Place We Call Redbird

In the spare bedroom of my home, there is a window that perfectly frames a sweet gum tree out back. It's like a living breathing picture of the seasons to be seen at your leisure. If you sit right next to the door, you can watch the lush green leaves of summer bake in the sun, or the orange leaves flirt with the wind as they glide to the ground in October. But my favorite is early spring. Watching the kelly-green buds poke their heads through the dead limbs as if they are waiting to see if the coast is clear to make their annual return. This room sat empty for a while, right after we first moved. Then it was a guest room, an art room, a junk room for the extra storage of things we didn't want to throw away yet. But once every few months, I would sneak into the space to see what it felt like at dusk. And at sunrise. I wanted to know how the light danced through the arms of the tree and left hieroglyphic shadows on the wall in the afternoon rays. I was curious to test how this room would breathe with someone actually living in it. The very first time I found out I was pregnant, I came into this room. I moved the boxes off the bed and shoved the pile of artwork I hadn't yet finished to the floor. I laid on my back to look out the window as the mid-morning light covered my legs. And for reasons I still don't understand, when I got the news my grandfather died, I ran into this room to cry out the window that I loved him. As if his soul made a pit stop in my backyard on the way to Glory.

About a year ago, my husband casually mentioned over dinner that he recently had several dreams about us adopting a child. This man, who never dreams, and if he does, he can't remember them by morning; was now sharing with me dreams that felt more like prophetic visions in the same tone he tells me about his golf game. In a familiar monotonous inflection, he told me of two more a few days later. I stood speechless each time with a flame of panic in my throat, because it was around that time that I, too, had dreams of adopting a son.

We stared at each other in a silent standoff, as if what we were about to discuss was so secretive that our walls and furniture couldn't even know. What better place to have a discussion such as that, but in the spare room? After careful consideration and several miles of pacing, we decided to start with fostering.

Over the next several weeks, we laid out our plan and began the process of becoming registered foster parents. In a pre-Covid world, this process would've been an in-person course that lasted three days. We would've met in a church basement in downtown Jackson, Mississippi, and listened to a social worker go through the logistics of raising a child that isn't yours and the horror stories of what those kids could've suffered. But being that we were in the dead center of 2020, all courses, lessons, and horror stories were now shared over *Zoom*.

The whole assembly was a bit more invasive than either of us had expected. The state wanted to know our history and childhood backgrounds. They needed to explore our incomes, how we fought, what church we went to, and if either of us had experienced sexual traumas. The questions leading up to our home study resembled more of an interrogation than an interview. We were becoming employees of the state, who would receive money per child, and as such we needed to get our fingerprints done at the local office of The Department of Human Services. I'd never been more thankful for a mask that day. The blue fabric covering my stunned mouth was a shield that I didn't know I would need. Our expedition to parenthood had taken quite the fall.

We had started off in crisp white offices of well-renowned experts in infertility. The local IVF specialist had his own interior designer stage the foyer comfortably so potential parents could relax. You could fall into tufted club chairs as they served tea and coffee and organic candy bars while a *Norah Jones* Pandora station echoed above. Nurses would pat you on the shoulder as you perused pamphlets of treatments that cost more than a semester at a state college. Those days of lab work and genetic surveys in spotless waiting rooms seemed like they happened in another life by that morning. We walked into a brown brick building that was hidden behind an old factory off the side of a highway and waited for a very overworked and underpaid social worker to call our names for fingerprints. I sat across from Kyle at a leaning card table with three legs and began to count the dead roaches that lay belly up in the corner.

Seven.

The blinds were dusty and hanging on by a thread as a hand-written poster on the adjacent wall reminded me to *smile at a stranger* that day. We knew that we lived in the poorest state with the most broken child welfare system in the country. The evidence of such statistics presented to us now over Zoom calls describing child molestation and disheveled state-run offices. I didn't feel above the situation, quite the opposite. We didn't consider ourselves too good for it. We were only collapsing with exhaustion at having made this decision so quickly, surprised at our arrival here. And terribly nervous for what was to come.

I cleared my throat to speak. "If someone had told me this is where we would end up, I wouldn't have believed them. If anyone had mentioned this to me years ago, I would have politely told them this is not for us. Kyle, what the hell are we doing here?"

He told me he wasn't sure. Our confidence was wavering, but none of our alarm bells were going off. Tears collected in the corner of my eyes just as the social worker returned our driver's licenses and social security cards. I tilted my chin towards my chest in an effort to hide my red face, once again thankful for the mask to hide most of my emotions. I was trying to understand the faith and strength that it would take for someone to take a child into their home, fall madly in love with them, feed them, hold them, and in a moment's notice—prepare to lose them. "Do you want to leave?" Kyle asked. I didn't. I wasn't wild about any of this. This foreign concept to procure a child through a government agency. The immediacy of taking in a child we don't know for an unknown amount of time. This wasn't the plan. This is not what I had dreamed of. But I knew in the pit of my stomach, we were exactly where we needed to be.

The steps unfolded for us pretty quickly over the next
several days. We were given a date for a home visit with our
social worker, and we had tons to do before then.

My spare room. The interchangeable guest room, art room,
junk room, and hoarder room now had to become a baby
room. We crammed the guest bed into the office, making it
feel like a shoebox dorm at college. We ordered a crib from
Target. The kind that can transform from an infant crib to a
twin bed, depending on what age we would receive.
We installed carbon monoxide alarms and hid baby food and
sippy cups in the back of our pantry. We did the best we
could in a short time and silently built a brick wall around
our marriage and hearts in an intrepid effort to not be
shattered by this process, which is known to be ruthless. The
Sunday arrived. We had the kindest and most thorough
social worker in the state, who cheerfully bounced through
our front door and began to take pictures of our home, even
the closets. She documented our floorplan, fire
extinguishers, and marriage license. Then, in a bashful
manner, she politely asked my husband and I to separate.

"I need to speak with you individually. I know it's a surprise
and uncomfortable, but if one of you could excuse yourself
first, I just have a few questions for each of you, and I don't
want you to monitor your answers for each other." Kyle took
our dog out to play as she penciled in her notes. She looked
up at me and smiled, then launched into some pretty
personal questions for a first-time meeting. Questions like
how we argue and makeup, who pays the bills, who does
most of the cooking, who has the worst temper, have we
ever seen a marriage counselor, do we like each other's
families.

"I hate asking just as much as you hate telling me, but you understand a child in state custody has seen and heard the worst. We just need to be sure we aren't taking them from one volatile home and placing them in another."

I understood. She continued, "What do you love most about your husband, do you trust him explicitly, could he be a good father?" I gave her the most honest, but uncharacteristically short answers I could. The state of Mississippi had pictures of all of my toilets, and now they were asking about the inner workings of my marriage. I wanted to keep my cards close to my chest, and I started to feel exposed in an unprotected way.

"Ok, Mr. Henry can come back in now. It's his turn."

I take pride in the fact that I return my grocery cart to the corral each trip, and I always pick-up trash on my morning walks. My moral compass has wavered over the years, but I consider myself a decent woman who knows the difference between right and wrong. But I vehemently knew that I was about to eavesdrop on my husband and the social worker. I couldn't help myself. I knew it was a low point. So was wearing Ugg boots with leggings and denim skirts, but I did that sad shit, too.

There are things you're just not supposed to hear. I know that now. There is a reason you're not in the room when people pray for you, or applaud you, or let down their guard for expressing how they truly feel about you. If we knew all of what was said on our behalf, good or bad, when we weren't within earshot, we would never leave the house.

Kyle answered the same questions as I had minutes before. He was gracious towards my cooking and matter of fact

about taking care of our finances. All of our answers
aligned.

But his last question was phrased differently than the one I'd
faced about him. She asked Kyle, *why* I would make a good
mother. To which he paused to consider his response. My
heart thumped in my ears as I leaned into the door of our
bedroom. My husband has quietly struggled with a stutter
since childhood. I couldn't know if his long pause was
thoughtful reflection, if he was making up a lie, or if he was
choking on a syllable. Silence broke as he painted me in a
much better light than I will ever deserve.

"She is the best person I know," he said. "She will be a
damn good mother, because she is a damn good woman."
My man of few words, simple and to the point.

I hid my emotions behind the unbelieved age-old excuse of
allergies, and we finished our home study by drawing a map
of our fire escape route if we had kids in the home.

Meet by the mailbox. That seemed like a solid plan. A few
days later we heard back from our social worker to let us
know that we'd been approved by the state and now the only
thing to do was wait for a call. "My supervisor did want me
to once again go over the difference between fostering and
adoption," she said.

Why?

She began to describe my bookshelf that stood next to the
window in the spare room. She couldn't help but notice the
teddy bear and family relics. Pictures of Kyle's grandmother
sat in pink frames that overlooked our collection of board
games on the lower shelves. "The room is so sweet," she

noted. But she was alarmed that it all seemed too personal. Too homey. Too familial. As if we were preparing for *our* child, not just *a* child.

"Most placements may not stay longer than a week, Mrs. Henry. They just need a warm bed and a stable home." I told her I had no problem knowing that a child would spend a night surrounded by family things. Our things. If I saw no issue with a child playing with the teddy bear that was handstitched by my great-grandmother, then the state of Mississippi should see no problem with it either.

"Wait, so they thought the room was too homey?" Kyle asked as I hung up the phone. I was crushed. "Are you kidding? How low is the bar set for foster children?" he asked.

Pretty damn low, it sounds like.

Two months before the room change and the home study, I was introduced to a woman who would quickly become one of my most treasured friends. Lindsey is tall and has an infectious laugh. Her dark hair makes her bright eyes shine in contrast and she is incredibly intelligent. She is a get-shit-done kind of woman who is known to study a menu days in advance so she has enough time to carefully consider her order. And she reminds me of my mother in a way that allows me to trust her with my life. Lindsey is a lobbyist. She works extremely hard to not be defined by her career, but when the legislature is in session, and her bills get passed, she is a sight for sore eyes. Lindsey and I fell into a new group of friends around the same time. And for the first time in my adult life, I had women around me who I didn't feel the need to compete with or hide from. Our little group bonded over our transparency on life and grief. Our cards were always on the table, face up. We challenged each other

in our successes and failures. Our goals and ideas, theologies
and politics. And we could cackle over our shared raunchy
sense of humor for hours on end.

Not long after adopting two children of her own from the
unforgiving foster care system, Lindsey pioneered a spiritual
retreat for women. The idea being that if you secluded
yourself into the mountains, with no phone service, no
makeup, no speaking, and if you choose, no eating; then you
could heal yourself of just about anything and settle
whatever you needed between you and God. The retreat was
based on a book called *The Gift of the Red Bird* by Paula
D'Arcy. The author documents her own retreat of solitude
after losing her child and husband in a brutal car crash. Paula
was so desperate to heal from her grief, she voyaged into the
Texas desert alone for four days with no food, little water,
and zero contact to the world, stripping herself of her senses
and bare necessities. Her only friend to guide her to healing
was a red cardinal. The story is very similar to *Wild* by
Cheryl Strayed, just without the heroin addiction.

Lindsey inviting me to this sacred retreat felt not only like a
huge honor, but an altar call I couldn't not answer. I had my
marching orders. For the weeks leading up to the retreat, I
would practice fasting, make sure I had hiking boots, and get
settled into the idea of not speaking. Like, at all.

The retreat couldn't have come at a better time. We had just
finished painting a crib for a child whose name I didn't
know and wasn't sure even existed. Kyle put the cradle
together, and as if we were in a choreographed routine,
handed me a paint brush as he put down the drill. His role
was to erect the fixture, while mine was to paint it and try
not to let my bitter anxiety get in the way of such a simple

task. I painted the crib a light shade of sage and tried not to fall in love with the idea of being a parent to a stranger.

I had not spoken much in the days prior to the retreat. I told myself that I was practicing for the vow of silence I would be taking, but that I think I was ready to not speak. I was growing exhausted of my own arrogant and negative thoughts, and I was counting down the minutes until not speaking was socially accepted, if not demanded. If you truly ever want to discover how entitled, spoiled, and greedy you are—I suggest you try one of these trips. There is no phone to distract or entertain you, no intrusive red notifications to shock you. No food or wine to fill you and take up space. No social status to protect you and no education to speak for you. You are you in the most modest sense. I found the idea of being stripped down, in nature, and mute, terrifying.

We made our way to Nauvoo, Alabama, and enjoyed one last meal before the fasting began. Four more women would join us the next day, already beginning their silences in the car on the way up. I'd never known a level of communal respect or self-assurance until I had to greet strangers in deafening silence. We nodded and pointed to the specified rooms and smiled awkwardly with our eyes. I observed these women who seemed to find their stride with such ease. They gracefully nodded and went straight to work praying and studying scripture by the fire. I was very out of my league.

The first full day of the retreat began with quiet time. Oh boy. The illustrious quiet time. I hadn't meditated in months and I knew the exact reason why.

I always find it a little insulting when people use time as a crutch.

Ugh, I wish I had time to meditate.

Oh please, I wish I had time for a manicure. A run. A lunch with a friend. A long bath. A...anything.

You do have time. You make time for what is important to you. Important *for* you. I could've made time to meditate leading up to the retreat, I just didn't because I was avoiding what the voice in my head was going to tell me. What the beat of my own heart would inform me in her pumping cadence. But now, in the middle of nowhere with about as much cellphone service to render my phone a calculator, I was forced to sit on a balcony that overlooked a lake and just *be*. I couldn't believe how difficult just sitting had become. Sitting and breathing and controlling your own thoughts. It was a test I had not studied for.

And it went something like this:

Ahh, okay. I can do this. Breathing in through the nose and out through the mouth. Find your rhythm of breathing. Rhythm. We will never be parents. Nope. That's negative and probably not true. Okay, back to breathing in rhythm, rhythm. Is Kyle going to leave me if I can't give him children? I'm not sure if I would blame him. He would be such a good father. My waking nightmare is him having an affair and then that woman being able to make him a father. No. Stop. Focus on rhythm breathing. Inhale for three...two...one. Exhale for three...two...one. Breathe in rhythm. It's just the rhythm of the niiiggght, oohh, ohhhh. Nope, that is from the Moulin Rouge soundtrack. Focus, my gosh, why is this so hard? Breathe. Expand your belly in deep breath. It is my brain, in my head. Control your thoughts. I can do this. Encouraging thoughts. I'm breathing fully. I'm safe. I'm blessed. I will accept motherhood in the

*means of which she will come to me, when she comes to me.
I'm thankful. I'm happy. What if we don't get approved to
foster? My body has rejected me four times now, what if the
state of Mississippi rejects us, too? I'm absolutely freaking
terrified. What if I'm just not meant to be a mother. I'm
starving. Is God mad at me? He is punishing me. Do
mountain lions live in Alabama? I don't know if I can ever
carry a child to full term. Tiger Woods is so talented. Ugh,
no. Focus on breathing. Steady your mind. I hope Britney
Spears is okay. Remember in junior high when you were
reading your science report in front of the class and snot fell
out of your nose? Oh my God.*

I was just about to throw in the towel on mastering the
neurotic sound of my inner thoughts, when Lindsey tapped
me on the shoulder and pointed up. It was time to hike.

We drove from our cabin around to the base point where the
path began. And as I heard the sharp crunch of leaves under
the tires, it hit me that I would have to hike behind Lindsey
the whole way and not be able to rely on her for comfort or
support in conversation. We were going to hike all day in
sheer quiet. We were halfway to our first break spot when I
realized I wasn't supposed to rely on Lindsey to comfort or
guide me through nature, I wasn't really even supposed to
rely on myself, all along I was supposed to be relying on
God. But she was right there in front of me, and I could talk
to myself in my head until I was blue in the face. How was I
supposed to lean on a God who I couldn't see or feel and
who I thought was punishing me with infertility?

Instead of surrendering to a God that I couldn't bring myself
to face, I chose instead, to focus on nature. And the scene
that was painted before me was one that would've hushed
me to a breathless quiet on any given day. The limestone
cliffs towered above us like skyscrapers. They were all

covered in a lime green moss that reminded me of my great-
aunt Mavis. She used to encourage us to use our
imaginations on nature walks when we were kids, and she
said moss was *where the fairies lived*. Wild ferns grew out
of cracks in the wall of mountainsides and a brook scuttled
through for miles and eventually rushed into a waterfall. The
stones tucked into the ravines were the size of SUVs and the
breeze carried a scent on its back that had me actually
finding the rhythm of deep breaths that I so craved that
morning. Lindsey would look over her shoulder to make
sure I was still behind her, and she kept pointing up. *Up?
How much further?* I felt like we were already twenty stories
high, but I could feel the altitude pulling, so further up we
went. My thoughts wandered toward the God that I was
forcing myself to ignore. He was certainly all around us. I
stood in His creation. I was climbing a mountain He told
where to stand, and yet every time I felt Him knock on the
door of my heart, I chose not to answer.

We do that so often in this life, don't we? We take our anger
out on God when the life He gave us doesn't go the way we
planned. There is a balance to be found in a walk with
Christ. I have found it, but not mastered it, and I'm not sure I
ever will. There is a line we walk that is cloaked in sin and
selfishness, hypocrisy and stupidity, grace and forgiveness.
As I struggled to follow Lindsey up the steep slope, my
selfish stupidity came rushing at me.

Reverence and obedience are two very different things.

Reverence and obedience are two very different things.

I am reverent, but I have never been obedient.

Ouch.

My thoughts were as shaky as my footing in the dry leaves. *I'm a child of God, hoping for a child of my own. Have I ever actually asked God for a child? Or did I just assume He would give me one? I'm so thankful that the people who went before me on this trail didn't move stones out of place. I need them to step over the meadow and the hanging branches to balance myself down the ravine. I'm so incredibly loved and loved well by my people and even God. How am I so loved and yet I forget that all the time. Do I actually allow myself to feel the love? No, I don't think I do.*

We made our way to a cliff that boasted an eleven-foot-tall cement cross. It had been there since the 1920's, and I was surprised to find that it was still very clean and sturdy. It had been well taken care of. *Reverence.*

Over the next two days we hiked and prayed, had quiet time and fasted. I made it forty-nine hours with no food. A personal record that I have no intentions to beat. I would turn my phone on to see if I had any missed calls or texts and laugh at myself for being so needy for connection to the world. Time passes very slowly when you are hungry, quiet, and secluded. My three-day trip felt more like weeks, and I was embarrassed to discover how much validation I needed from a phone.

I couldn't get the idea of reverence and obedience out of my head, so I figured I could start with something small. On our last day, I knew I wanted to challenge myself on being alone with God in nature. I cherish my alone time. I love being in the great outdoors. But combining the two and being alone in the mountains is usually where I draw the line. I'm no good at directions and have few survival skills that would come in handy if I were to stumble upon an avalanche or a mountain lion. But I was desperate for a kind of respite that only comes with quiet self-exploration. As I was journaling and praying before my lone walk in nature, visions of me having to fight off a bobcat were playing on a loop in my head. I was just about to chicken out and stay safe on the balcony when a voice told me to go now.

I rationalized it and told myself that I would walk around the cabin, but the voice persisted.

Why are you going to the road when I've called you to the lake?

Reverence is different than obedience.

So, I gathered all the courage I possessed and started towards the lake. I took slow careful steps down the hill and kept an eye out for snakes even though it was November and freezing. I paced myself as I made my winding turns through to the lake and remained silent when I saw deer tracks in the mud. *Shit. How do you fight off a buck? Are they aggressive? Do deer charge at their prey. Do deer have prey? If I see a buck, I will just lie down so he can run me over.*

It was so quiet on the lake that my ears were ringing, and the water was so still I swore that I was looking at glass. And for the first time since we arrived, actually for the first time ever in my life, I surrendered.

I inhaled deeply and the wind carried that same sweet scent from the hike. It was a pure fragrance that I think we don't notice in our day-to-day lives but it is always there. Nature is one of the best gifts from God. And still, we choose blinding screens filled with futile personas over sunsets time and time again. I looked up to where the clouds met the treetops, and I felt a familiar attitude greet me.

Okay, God. Here I am. I was obedient. I'm here at the lake. I'm alone, just like you wanted me. Now what? Show me what you wanted me to see.

It was not my proudest moment, because here is the thing — God owes us nothing. Zilch.

I'm no biblical scholar, but I'm pretty sure nowhere in the Bible does is say, "Do one tiny thing for God and He will entertain you." Nor does it say, "If you step out on faith and prepare a room for a child you're not carrying, God will give you one as a prize."

I sat on the boat dock and felt shame with nowhere to hide. The idea of an empty nursery in my home filled me with just as much hope, as it did embarrassment.

A Tolkien quote came to mind. *A divine punishment is also a divine gift.* In an interview several years ago, Stephen Colbert referenced this quote and translated the idea as *what of these gifts aren't of God*, when discussing the death of his own father and brothers.

What we see as punishment, could be the best gift. What we see as a disaster, could be the genesis of who we are meant to be. Either way, nothing comes to us that is not of God. Nothing is outside of His hand.

I had to thank God for my infertility and then give it back to Him, but I wouldn't. He wanted me to lay down my burdens right there on the dock.

"But it's mine," I cried aloud.

My voice cracked and my tongue felt stiff as I broke my silence. *But this is mine.* My infertility. My grief. It's mine to hold and spew my anger on. It's mine to figure out and fix. It's mine to use as a shield. It's mine. I can't give it up or lay it down, because then...well, then it couldn't hurt me anymore. If I didn't cling to my losses, I would truly have nothing left to hold on to.

Nothing but Him.

The potential names of children I'd been storing in my heart were becoming harder to remember as I questioned if I was meant to be a mother at all. Remembering back to a night that felt like a lifetime ago, when I cried myself to sleep, demanding that God take away my desire to be a mother. I was toying with the idea of full surrender when I heard leaves rustling and footsteps from behind me. Panic jolted through my body like a lightning rod, and I was paralyzed in fear. This was it. I was going to be mauled to death by a raccoon. I looked over my shoulder to see a sweet older fisherman smiling gently at me. In a reverence for my solitude, he stopped to watch me on the dock and waited for me to motion that he could join me. In a selfish assumption, I again waited for a cloud-parting and shocking message from God to speak through the gentlemen to me, which of course, never came. Small talk about the weather was exchanged, and I wished him luck with the fish as I started back towards the cabin.

I made my way back through the same trail and found that I was relieved to have not had some epiphany from God. There is no need to receive all the answers at once. We don't need all the answers at once. He doesn't owe me an explanation for my flaws or grief. Life is a continued slow dance of hushed yeses with Him. We continue to work on saying yes to Him, which will always be better than saying yes to self. That lesson is to be learned day after day after day.

Our trip ended on an overcast Sunday and by the time I got home, the sweet gum tree that could be viewed from the spare room was changing her colors under the autumn air once again. Another season was coming to a close, and another was just beginning. After I unpacked my luggage and kissed my husband who I missed way too much, I made my trusted al dente pasta with butter and crushed pepper and cozied up to the idea of waiting in grief and not expecting anything from it.

I scanned the spare room and sank down next to the door, once again to soak in the tree, and the empty crib, and the seasons, and the waiting. A peaceful stillness stirred over me and I knew that the room would sit empty for a while. A long while. Kyle came up behind me to close the door, and as he smiled at me, I realized that I was actually breathing in perfect rhythm.

6

And Away We Go

My grandmother had an older sister who was eighteen years her senior. In my experience, siblings with that large of an age gap usually don't have a close bond, but somehow Mavis and Faye did. Their mother, my great-grandmother, was a soft-spoken seamstress who hand-rolled fresh biscuits from scratch every morning and sewed her own clothes most of her life, not wearing a store-bought dress until she was in her fifties. My grandmother was the youngest of five and adored all of her siblings, but she held a rare closeness with her big sister. My great-aunt Mavis was a pistol. She left her hometown of Sylacauga, Alabama, just before World War II and traveled to California to be a dancer and then came back across the country to Panama City, Florida, to find work. She worked in night clubs and casinos selling packs of cigarettes, cigars, and playing cards to customers, who were mostly intoxicated men. She had very little money during that time, but I recall her telling my grandfather once that she *used what she had to get by*, if you know what I mean.

She would tell my mom and her sisters that she was a movie star, and they believed her for longer than they probably should have. Mavis had eyes that were so blue, they almost looked white, and I firmly believe we all inherited our filthy senses of humor from her. She lived life in the fast lane for the daughter of a Baptist music minister. She was beautiful and creative and had a wild streak that would make grown men blush. She and my grandmother shared inside jokes and dance routines they would perform in the front yard, well into their seventies and eighties.

Not long after my grandparents passed away, I found a picture of Mavis standing on the beach.

She had thick legs and a small waist, and she was holding a cigarette between her index and middle finger. She looked into the camera as if she was holding one hundred secrets behind her smirk. I turned the picture over and realized she was thirty years old the day the snapshot was taken. Thirty was old in 1941. She was unmarried and had no goals of settling down and would never have children of her own. I don't think I've ever wanted to know why so badly until I had issues of my own in that department. I've wondered if she couldn't, or if she just didn't want to. My grandmother asked her one time why she and her first husband never had kids. To which she responded, "well because we never..." you can fill in the rest.

In the picture she looked happy. Not a temporary fleeting happiness, but almost an arrogant joy. It appeared she lacked for nothing. Not love or lust, not friendship or a tan. In that moment, she had all she would ever need because she had already taken it with force.

When I think about what life was like in those days, I feel lightheaded with jealousy. Wages were low, but so was the cost of living. Families seemed closer and homes were always ready for friends to drop by, because *dropping by*

was something people actually did back then. The pictures I
have of my people in the good ole days paint a tale of things
actually being good. Sure, there was a world war, and
everyone had their issues, but overall, I believe they had it a
little better than we do now. People made jokes because they
actually wanted to be funny, not because they wanted to go
viral. Pictures were taken to hold on to memories and not to
hold attention for likes or fame. People appreciated all they
had because they could remember a time when they had
nothing at all.

Times were simple, but the people were not.

In the same box that I found the picture, I also found a letter.
Oddly enough, Mavis wrote it to my grandmother on
February 8, 1962. My grandmother would take her last
breath on February 8, 2019, a detail I can't name as just a
coincidence. I read the letter as I sat on the floor of my
grandfather's study. Boxes surrounded me with old papers
and pictures, family relics and Sear's catalogs from the
sixties. I must have read the letter ten times in a row, finding
a new fact and emotion each time that I scanned it over. I
tried to remember what her voice and vivacious laughter
sounded like as I soaked in each word.

And this is what she said, verbatim.

———————————

*Dearest Dattie Tae, Sweet William, Necie Bug, and Rolly
Polly Sugar Pot:*

*I send each of you a gallon of hugs and a pinch on the
bottom. I hope the youngerns are over the pocks and measles
and are well and happy again. Our little mother knows how
to look after her little ones, so I will look after you! I don't*

*know how I have waited this long to be with my bosom pal
again, except that I have a brain to think over past good
times and keep glad inside by just remembering. At times, I
laugh out loud just thinking about usses. The rediculous has
always been funny to me. And even this spelling is funny, but
just know what I mean.*

*I enjoyed being at home this past weekend very much.
Mamma and I got in the car and did what we wanted to and
didn't let Ressie hold us back. She was doing what she
wanted to do and as you know, it was the same with her. She
met me really in form. She knew I was coming a week before
I got there and had that long to prepare. I don't know why it
is that she can't stand to be around me sober? The only way
she can take me is by getting loopy to forget. I have been
working on this real hard to see why after all these years
that I affect her this way. And I think the answer is finally
coming to me, thank goodness.*

In my trying to help her, I've driven her away.

*In trying to show her how I feel she is running from what I
have. In my humbleness, she has seen hysteria, instead of
confidence. I am going to change my way of doing and quit
trying to show her as she thinks I am bossing her and resents
this, as she is 50 years old. All these years I have loved her
so much and wanted her to be happy, but until she finds this
for herself, I am only driving her away from me. You have
shown me how to overcome this, my bosom pal. You have
enjoyed life at home in spite of her. You have had your
friends come in and not let what she does hamper you and
that has been the thing to do.*

*Thank goodness, Mamma and I are turnin' her aloose in this
way too.*

*We went to town and Mamma wanted to send Necie a
present cause she had been sick, and she had a good time
buying it. This made Mamma happy. She said she doesn't
know why but she is partial to Necie and she can't help it. I
said "Mamma, you are only human. And don't be ashamed
to admit that you love one child over another." I feel the
same way about some people. She wanted to send Diane
something just cause she did Necie, but I said she was too
little to know if she got anything or not and her day is
coming too. Mama is collecting cotton to piece both of them
a quilt. How glad I am that she will be doing something she
loves to do and that it is for your sweet girls.*

*We went to church Sunday and she wore her new hat and
blouse and her beads and ever was she pretty. We went to
see grandma over at Ava's Saturday night and enjoyed
seeing Ava talk with her new teeth in. She can really put on.
I had a big laugh looking at Ressie mock her. You can
imagine how it must've looked to see Ressie, half drunk and
making fun of Ava gritting her false teeth. I laughed until I
cried. Ressie had been over to see Morris and came back
holding on to the fence. I couldn't even bear to look at her
come in. Ressie told us about seeing an old man at the curb
market with a long beard. She told him he looked like the
Devil himself. I said "Mamma, I wonder if he had a tail and
red horns and wore a red suit?" I suppose that is what
Ressie thinks the devil looks like. But I now know there is no
such thing as a devil that looks like that. I guess I got the
idea from the Red Devil Lye we use to make soap.*

*I tried to assure Mamma that God wasn't going to put Ressie
in a fiery pit and burn her up cause she didn't do just like we
think she should. And I think Mamma is willing to put her in
God's hands, knowing I feel that she can trust him to take
care of her. And he isn't going to hurt her. Mamma wouldn't*

do this, so why should we think that a God who knows more about us than a human father knows, do such a thing? We tell too much of the parables without understanding the parables. God is love. And he understands why Ressie or I do the things we do, and he loves us in spite of our unworthiness. I used to be so afraid to say anything like this, but I'm not anymore because I see it in a different light.

When you have time read the enclosed. I gave this lecture to 50 church ladies on Monday night and we had a wonderful meeting. The topic was "The Meaning of Suffering" it has taught me many things. None of us are above suffering, are we?

Howard just left after lunch and the news said that Jane Mansfield was on Coral Island and had been stuck under a boat and the sharks were after her. I told Howard I guess one of her big titties came out of her swimsuit and was floating by and she thought it was a shark! He said it must've been too, as there are no sharks in that water!

Aunt Ilene and Uncle Blair are parting ways. She said at Christmastime she couldn't afford him. I said maybe he will straighten up and fly right? She said, "All I want him to do is straighten up and fly out!"

Howard said she married him for the sex and money, so I guess she wasn't seeing either, or else she would be satisfied! She wrote to me yesterday and said he had been gone since January 18th. She has a new car and Oliver wants her to come visit him in Europe. Also, she said she had talked to Blair and he wants her to change her mind, but she said, "I don't think I will!"

We are invited to do lots of things this month. Howard will speak to the Kiwanis club on the 21st and the Sunday school

students this month. I will give my same lecture on
"Suffering" on the 30th of March to another church here in
town. I already spoke to them at Christmastime and I've
been invited again!

I like my boss more and more. You know this heavenly
influence is good for me. He is kind and thoughtful, good.
And I am completely happy in my job.

Write to me my love and take good care of everyone and
yourself. I hope all is well with you all. Just a card will
make Mamma happy, she is getting old and needs petting.

She loves you all so much and I don't blame her. I do
toooooooo.

Your bosom pal forever.

All my love,
Lou.

According to my mother, *Dattie Tae,* was a nickname that
Mavis called my grandmother. Her name was Mary Faye,
but a neighbor who liked to hit the moonshine a bit too hard
and too often, would slur as he said hello, slushing her name
instead to Dattie Tae. As you can imagine, in fits of laughter,
the name stuck. Ressie was their other older sister. She was a
nurse in the first world war who became addicted to pain
killers after having easy access to them in the hospitals. I'd
heard from my mom and aunts that Ressie was an addict
who battled esophageal cancer and couldn't speak clearly or
eat solid foods for close to a decade. My mother vividly
remembers an occasion where Mavis and her mother had to
physically restrain Ressie in an effort for her to not ingest
any more pills. Even with this information, I still thought

that people who lived in simpler times must have had
simpler problems.

But as proven, each generation has their own turmoil.

At some point in the late 1940's, Mavis began her walk with
the man from Galilee. I wish I knew for certain what caused
her revival, but I suppose the why of it doesn't matter. Either
way, the Mavis who took us on nature walks to hug trees,
thank the stars, and point out where the fairies lived, could
also quote scripture at the drop of a hat, and she dedicated
the rest of her working days to her church and telling others
about Jesus. Not much changed about her after her baptism.
She somehow became even more of a bright light. She still
loved a colorful curse word and a good sex joke, but she
never touched alcohol ever again. I guess one day she looked
around and saw that drinking had not given her much to hold
on to. She was the daughter of an alcoholic, the sister of two
alcoholics, she would eventually marry an alcoholic—and
again, I thought she had it easy.

I thought they all did.

Mavis had an extraordinary flare for life. She curated the
most beautiful collection of costume jewelry in the south and
after many years as a widow, she married her high school
sweetheart at the age of seventy-seven. She relished in
nature and had the most beautiful garden in all of Sylacauga.

By the time I was in middle school, Mavis was in her late
eighties. Her health declined pretty rapidly after Alzheimer's
set in. But before the disease stole what was left, my
grandparents took my cousins and me on a summer trip to
Alabama to see Mavis. She was the first person I'd ever
known in my life to be completely secure and sound in who
she was. She would greet her loved ones, and sometimes

even strangers, with these wide armed open hugs and melodic laughter. She would hold your hands while she asked you questions that she genuinely wanted answers to. And she would see straight through you with her piercing eyes. She would make jokes and tell outlandish stories, and she wasn't afraid of others' opinions.

The very essence of this woman was like a firework show over a calm lake. Peaceful and exciting, all at once.

No matter how much time had passed, they fell back into the same conversation with laughter and easy stride. Mavis and Faye were cooking dinner in her small kitchen while my grandfather sipped his scotch and us kids explored her garden. I watched from the window as two sisters moved as one throughout the space. They exchanged seasonings and knives without skipping a beat over conversation and then would snicker at each other with winks and tickles. It had never occurred to me before, that some of your best friends can be found inside your own family. And that is what they were, the very best of friends.

There was a show on CBS called *The Jackie Gleason Show* back in their day. The theme song was called *And Away We Go* and the host, Jackie Gleason, would do a little move where he would twist his waist and cock up a leg as his opening monologue ended and he would say, and awayyyy weeee goooooo. And that is how he kicked off each show.

I wish I could've been a fly on the wall the first time they mimicked the move, but for the next fifty years, before one sister would get in the car to leave the other, they would stand in the front yard or driveway singing the lyrics and kicking up their own legs. As our summer trip to Mavis' ended that year, they did the move as my cousins and I watched in embarrassment, afraid a neighbor would see us and somehow report back to all of our friends at home. They laughed at their lack of balance and needed to hold on to one another as they swung a leg up.

We hugged Aunt Mavis goodbye and climbed into the van to make our way home to Mississippi. My memory of these two sisters and friends embracing on a steep hill is one I don't think of as often as I should. As the van pulled away, Mavis stayed in the driveway singing and waving and blowing kisses to us until we were out of her sight. With tears in her eyes, my Mamaw looked in the rearview mirror and said, "She sure is something, isn't she?"

Yes ma'am. She sure was.

7

A Long December

There is an unmistakable sound that can erupt from the chest of a human. It is a primal roar that comes from the deepest part of a being and once you've heard it, you can immediately recognize the pitches of anguish. It's the sound of grief bellowing from the mouth in inaudible surges, as the air gets thicker to breathe. This emotion rising from deep within your belly, is like having your body be taken over by a foreign entity. And while the mysterious emotion of grief pulsates through your system, the world will see you as unsteady.

The thing about grief is that no one can really explain to you how to maneuver through the waves of terror that will make you feel like you're drowning. It is impossible for someone to sit you down and say, "Hey, when the worst of the worst happens to you, this is how you handle it, and how you will feel, and how you can behave." There is no dress rehearsal for grief.

A dull pain will creep up through your lower back and make a camp in your belly for months on end, as you navigate life

in darkness. Life will start to feel riddled with stings of hurt
and emptiness. These feelings of grief will shock you in their
briefness and slowly dissipate like a limb regaining blood
flow after falling asleep. But the stubborn pride of us, all of
us, would have one believe that grief holds no bounds on us.
You think you're tougher than that. Stronger than sadness.
Your brain will trick you into thinking that you're stronger
than crying in the pharmacy.

You're better than the nothingness of sitting in a quiet car
for thirty minutes after you've parked and killed the ignition.
But when you arrive at the place of sadness and grief. And
you look up to find that you're no better than the lost people
you used to judge in your free time. You settle on the idea of
your own numbness.

Grief is transformative in her crest. The salt water of waves
gulps you up in one sitting and leaves you gagging on your
own tears. *Breathing, two, one. Exhale, two, one.*

Grief is the unspeakable emotion. It makes us
uncomfortable. Uncomfortable to live in and uncomfortable
to watch and discuss. Your neighbors will talk about you if
they don't agree with the way you handle it, and your friends
will rush you into survival mode, so they don't have to
suffer alongside you. Grief is a black blanket that you don't
wish to be wrapped in. Covering you entirely and only
releasing you on its own free will. The worst part of being
under grief's covers is that you don't want to be seen, but
under her veil is a spotlight with your name on it. People see
you more clearly now that you have dark circles under your
eyes, and you're balancing on the tight rope of wanting to be
forgotten and wanting to be coddled.

We grieve for all different sorts of things. We grieve for the
loved ones we lost. We grieve for loved ones who hurt, the

ones we can't help. We grieve ideas that never came to fruition, and we grieve a future we dreamt of that never came to pass. All of this is allowed.

All of it is different, but the same. And all of it weaves together the fabric of who we are.

We concoct coping mechanisms that are just as surprising to us as they are the people watching. I, for one, faced grief with a sudden shopping addiction and a deep hunger for a good argument. Both cruxes colliding a few years ago around Christmas. It was the same year that I had two miscarriages five months apart. This was on the tail of losing both grandparents, two other pregnancies, and me having watched my sister bury her own daughter. By that point, grief was an old friend that I'd greet in the shower each morning.

But my husband shines during Christmas. He is in his element eating frozen Oreo balls and watching holiday movies starting in November. That Christmas, Kyle was particularly convicted about giving back. We'd joined a new church and he wanted to do his part for the *Angel Tree* giving project. My grief made me angry and bitter; but in an effort, to avoid his own grief, he did his best to brush everything under the rug and become *Kris Kringle*. We...He picked an angel from the tree weeks in advance. Kyle kept the yellow ticket with the child's information in his truck, and I would pretend to not see it on the way to church. Each Sunday leading up to the holiday season our priest would remind us that *Angel Tree* gifts are due two weeks before Christmas and to keep the presents unwrapped.

He would remind me each week that we needed to go shopping to get the items for the child, a three-year-old girl.

She was tiny. They marked her sizes at *2T* and all she
wanted was a Minnie Mouse battery powered electric car. I
asked for one more week, playing it off as if I was busy, but
I knew he could see my end game. I wanted him to forget
about it. I wanted to ignore it. I wanted to spend the money
on myself, to lick my wounds, and go home with a bottle of
red wine.

He stared at me with a look that said, "I see you, and I
respect you, but you're not winning this one." So, off to
Wal-Mart we went. Kyle had searched the internet for the
Minnie Mouse car and found that Wal-Mart was the only
carrier. I avoid Wal-Mart most days out of the year anyway,
but certainly I have the smarts to avoid it like the plague
around the holidays. The store was crowded and rushed. It
seemed the whole town had the same idea we did that day. I
grabbed a shopping cart and said, "We should probably start
with the car first and then go get the clothes." I had no idea
how big the boxes are for those little cars. It barely fit into
the buggy and I couldn't see over the box to steer our way
throughout the isles.

I was fine. I was on auto pilot and tunnel visioned my way
through the store. I was online shopping in my head on what
I would be treating myself with for having gone through this.
We turned the isle to make our way to the clothes section
when we passed a family. The young red headed boy
followed his parents through the isle as he adjusted his black
rimmed glasses to take a better look at us. "Wow, their
daughter sure is lucky," he said brushing his hands over the
box in our cart. My voice cracked as I called out to Kyle. His
hand found my lower back and he said, "I know. I heard
him, too."

He didn't mean to crush me. The little boy with flaming hair
was making a precious comment and he wasn't wrong.

Some kid was very lucky that year, she just wasn't our kid. I
cried across the store and Kyle kept telling me to go sit in
the truck. Through tears I chuckled and asked him if he
knew how to put together an outfit for a little girl? He smiled
at me and said he could've figured it out. I drew my focus on
matching leggings to sweaters, and socks to hair bows. The
boys voice on repeat in my mind as his comment cut deeper
and deeper.

On the way home we decided to go on and get a tree. "I will
go ahead and start decorating the living room, and you can
work on that," I pointed to the pink box in the bed of his
truck.

Being shoved into celebrating felt like I was standing in a
crowded room begging for someone to help me, and no one
cared to look up.

In the same way most arguments and short tempers meet
their match around that time of year, mine too, began with
colorful language as I cursed my way through untangling
Christmas lights. I threw the ball of lights down on the
ground and made my way to the garage to yell at Kyle for
not having braided the strands properly eleven months ago. I
flung open the back door and was greeted by a sight that I'd
prayed for, but not like this. I'd lost hours of days dreaming
about what it would be like to be a parent on Christmas.
Playing Santa and watching a child marvel at twinkle lights
for the first time. The dream always being postponed, one
season more. The wind was kicked out of my chest as I
registered what I saw.

There was my husband hard at work. He had his toolbox
open and wrenches of all sizes laid at his feet. The pink
convertible was on its head as he screwed in the music box

that could play as it drove. I watched him as he meticulously read each step and executed them perfectly. Kyle is a textbook rule follower. Bouts of jealously came over me in waves as he studied the instruction manual with such care.

He cared.

And in that moment, I found it exhausting to care about anything at all. *Why? Why? Why am I going through this? Why is this happening to us? And why was he so slap-shit happy about buying a toy for a kid, and we couldn't even give it to her ourselves?* In my heartbroken rage I launched into him and berated him for the tangled lights. I told him the house stunk and the heat wasn't working. I told him to not come inside until I was ready for his help. I may have seen spots and called him every name under the sun except a child of God. The illness of grief that turns into rage will leave you intoxicated.

Kyle turned to look over his shoulder at me, and I'm sure he saw a two-headed demon instead of his bride. My voice rattled with expletives, and pointless demands. Like a child who'd not gotten her way, I slammed the door and waited for his apology. The apology he didn't owe me. I huffed back inside to pick up the ball of tangled Christmas lights and could suddenly see the zip tie that held it together. I heard the backdoor open, and I looked up to see a stunned husband walking on eggshells to approach his bitch wife. Without saying a word, he pulled out his pocketknife and cut the zip tie, freeing the lights of their web in one swoop.

He wasn't taking my bait.

He wasn't poking or snapping back.

And then I could feel it. The raging howl came up from my belly in a final effort to give my soul something to grind against. "Fight with me. Why won't you fight back, damnit? Give me something to feel," I roared at my spouse. My words pelted and stung him, but he just stood there and let me break under my own grief. He slowly started to speak, reminding me that fighting just to fight, just to have something to feel and focus on, isn't something we do.

"Do you want me to take the car and clothes back?"

"Of course not. You did a good thing, don't let me spoil it."

I sat on the floor and could feel the needles of the Frazier Fir sting my legs. Kyle squatted down in front of me and took my chin into his hand. I asked him if he was sad at all, because he sure didn't look it to me. But that is the thing about sadness; just because mine was so recognizable, accompanied by anger, didn't mean that Kyle's was insignificant. He was sad, too. And checking off all the holiday boxes was his way. His Band-Aid. He went back out to finish up the car, and I started trimming extra branches from the tree to make my mantel garland. Every few minutes I would walk over to the backdoor to say I was sorry. So truly sorry. And my gracious husband told me it was okay.

We took our time decorating the tree and the living room. I told the same stories that I've told him every year of our marriage about why I love the teacup ornament from England, and how my dad sprinkled powdered sugar around his boots to make it look like Santa's footprints. I stared at the nativity scene for a long time, and carefully placed the ceramic *Dicken's Village* homes that we inherited from Kyle's grandmother on the sofa table. Each year as we decorate, we pick a Christmas movie to play in the

background. That year, we only played low music and let
steam from our fight, my fight, aerate and clear the room.

We continued our way through another Christmas season
filled with Oreo balls and presents, pregnancy
announcements on social media, and pity hugs from
relatives. When the day finally came for us to drop off the
car and clothes to our church, Kyle told me I didn't have to
go with him. I ignored him and climbed in the truck anyway.

I carefully laid the three outfits I'd picked out on a table, and
Kyle parked the pink convertible next to it. My grief
subsided as I looked around the fellowship hall and saw our
priest marvel at how many bicycles, toys, and clothes had
been provided. Good deeds done in earnest; blessings
provided by people who were just as crushed as me, but they
were somehow more capable of giving than I was. A spark
of anger flickered within me, and I quickly smothered it
down. I wondered if most of the people I'd come in contact
with in my life, who I'd classified as jerks, or rude, or
assholes, or just down right mean—I wondered what they
were grieving, too.

That year, I took down the decorations on Christmas Eve. In
hindsight, I had no business putting up a tree at all. When we
need to take breaks and sit things out, we need to remember
to give ourselves permission to do that. If you can't find it
within you to celebrate, don't.

We need to remember that while grief is a house guest, it's
hard to entertain anyone else.

I was itching to do my beloved end-of-the-year routine. The
week between Christmas and New Year's, I deep clean the
house, get everything organized, buy new candles, and fill in
my planner for the coming year.

I sat at my spotless dining room table as candles burned in each room of the house. A powerful sense of relief fell over me as I penciled in birthdays and anniversaries in my planner and smiled. "Finally, a new year, and I just know it will be better than last year."

Ah yes, 2020 would be the best year yet.

8

The One Where Everyone Is Pregnant

After four miscarriages, you start to understand that your personal view of parenthood is quite rare. My husband and I could stand in the middle of the road, with our feet firmly planted in two very different camps. On one side, we were fortunate enough to know what a pregnancy announcement felt like. The joy and congratulations, the fear and excitement, and the fall-on-your-face, pinch-me-I-am-dreaming, this-is-what-life-is-all-about love. And on the other side—we know what it's like to escape the jaws of parenthood by the skin of our teeth, pinching yourself in disbelief that you will be able to sleep for eight interrupted hours one more night and sustain your sanity without *Paw Patrol* making you its bitch.

It's a constant back-and-forth dance of wanting so desperately to be a parent in one second and then in the other being smug about having a pristine white couch. These emotions are not independent from each other and can change on a whim. Deep down we knew we desperately

wanted to be parents but were still confused as to why we'd
been given so many false starts.

After a whirlwind 2020 that shook every human of every
nation to their core, the south experienced an ice storm of
biblical proportions. Our humble home state of Mississippi,
which usually experiences weather so humid that you can
expand two sizes under the August sun, was now surviving
single digit temps and inches of ice and snow in February.
We took it as an opportunity for respite after a weird 2020
came to a close.

Like the universe was saying, "One more week in your
homes. Cozy up next to the fire and just be." But the
southern folk that we are, we looked at a once in a lifetime
snowstorm as our playground for the week. Kyle and I
turned into kids as soon as we stepped out the front door.
Throwing balls of ice at each other, flinging boiling water
into the air to watch it hit the ground as a powder, and using
old cookie sheets as sleds. We were waddling like penguins
on ice down our street, laughing until we cried at the
numbness in our fingers, when I looked up to realize we
were the only homeowners on our street with no children.

Neighbors stood on the sidewalks to film their kids sliding
and sledding down the hill on wake boards that were
intended for July use only. Kyle went about his way,
unscathed as he turned over his shoulder and said, "Man this
is awesome. I feel like a kid again." To which I responded,
"This makes me want to try for kids again."

I suddenly felt foolish and misplaced on our busy street of
ice skaters. How many more ice storms would we have to go
through without kids? How many more Christmases would
seem frivolous without the excitement of a child ripping

open a gift from Santa on Christmas morning? How many more Halloweens would we face answering the door for other people's dinosaurs and superheroes? Celebrations were getting harder to celebrate. I stood in the kitchen to ask Kyle how he felt about all of this, as I pointed out to him that it was almost two years since our last loss. Still stunned that this was happening to us and being too scared to go back to the doctor for more testing, the boiling water started to pour over the stove as he answered me.

"I know I want kids. And I thought we would've had them by now, but babe, I'm selfish."

I turned off the stove eye to listen more clearly.

"I love our life and our marriage. I love our freedom of time and finances. I'm selfish and I love the way our life is now. And I know I want more out of life, but I also want more time with you, just us two."

I jumped into his arms and began sobbing before he could finish his sentence. He said what I was afraid to admit. For the last few years, I'd felt as if life was passing us by. All of our closest friends were on their second or third children, while we still had none. We were stuck in the place of being embarrassed at our failed attempts and ashamed of our prolonged selfishness, both places feeling safe from commitment.

We knew that in life, there is no better feeling than to love and raise a child. But we also knew that some of our friends rushed into it and had several boxes of goals left unchecked the day they became parents. To quote one of my favorite authors, Elizabeth Gilbert, "Having a baby is like getting a tattoo on your face. You really need to be certain it's what you want before you commit."

Please, please, tattoo my face. Just not right now.

With each loss we felt like we'd been robbed and rescued all at once, and for a long time I didn't allow myself the space to feel those conflicting emotions.

I always thought I would stumble into motherhood. A whoopsie-daisy of fate was going to push me down the hill of "Uh oh, well we weren't planning for this, but I'm pregnant!" I'd never known anyone who actually had to try to get pregnant, and if they did fight for it, they didn't talk about it. All I'd ever witnessed was well-timed conceptions or teenage accidents. I figured my story would develop in a more *laissez-faire* light, something like...

dream sequence harp music

I would meet a man. A very rich, independently wealthy (think tech and Bitcoin), handsome man. Not the textbook handsome, but like the *he has a mysterious scar on his cheek from an accident in his rough past,* handsome. We would meet and have a whirlwind romance and then through a totally surprising, *ohmigod I don't believe it,* revelation I would fall pregnant even before he proposed, which he would obviously still do because he was crazy about me. And *tah-dah!* That is how I would become a mother.

We would exchange vows on a beach as the sun set. In Fiji. With our yacht floating in the distance. My small belly showing under my effortlessly chic chiffon gown. And that would be it. My happily ever after.

I'm cackling at my own stupidity.

But why did I even consider that storyline to begin with?

BECAUSE HOLLYWOOD HAS MADE BILLIONS
TELLING ME THAT HORSESHIT LIE.

You've seen it. *Knocked Up*, the last scene of *Notting Hill*,
Nine Months, Look Who's Talking, Look Who's Talking Too,
and *Baby Boom*. They all made it look easy and quick. At
least the getting pregnant or getting a baby part. There is no
struggle or loss, no effort, and no financial woes in those
storylines.

My real story actually played out like this.

I met a really handsome guy in college. The normal and
even shy kind of handsome. He was so broke that he worked
four jobs at once and had never been on a yacht. We met,
began dating, fell in love, moved in together, financially
struggled, moved cities, lived with his parents, got married,
hated our jobs, gained a ton of weight, went through a
significant amount of loss, trauma, and depression, and then
realized that getting pregnant and having a human child is
actually really hard work.

And they lived happily ever after.

For the last three years of our marriage, I've made
intentional decisions to align our life for parenthood. The car
we bought, the house we bought, and even the job I chose—
it was all to make our future a little easier with kids. We
bought one of the safest cars on the road and have yet to
strap a car seat in the back. It's like altering your life to
prepare for a hurricane that changed directions in the gulf.

Not long ago, we had dinner with a couple of dear friends.
They of course, were parents themselves. The same people

who used to marvel at movies, concerts, job promotions, and day-drinking on Saturdays, were now supremely happy describing how their daughter stuck English peas in her nose and every electrical socket in the house. I couldn't believe the discussion at dinner was how to carefully use a pair of tweezers to pull peas out of a child's nose. And the punchline? They all laughed until they cried because smooshed peas are the same color as boogers. As my friend retold us the story, her tears from laughter almost turned to tears of joy. Every friend I have who is a parent, is exhausted. They usually smell weird. They aren't sleeping, they are running on fumes, and they feel like they are failing all the time, but they are all blindly and breathlessly happy.

Happiness is fleeting, isn't it? Happiness is like a scent that you stumble into and tugs on a memory. Like walking outside and hitting an air pocket of honeysuckle, or a grill burning on a summer night. When I turned thirty, my husband kept pressuring me about what I wanted for a gift. It took months of me convincing him that all I wanted was a party, no gifts, just a party. We invited friends to the house and had way too much food and wine, and I felt entirely grown up. I stood in my bathroom touching up my face with powder and I could hear my closest friends laughing in my living room. I reapplied my lipstick and took a sip of wine as I walked back towards the party. I could see my best friend from childhood talking to friends from college as Kyle brought in another round sausage off the grill and in that moment, I thought, "It doesn't get any better than this." Buckets of my happiness were found in moments of that evening.

After my third loss, I wandered over to the *TTC* side of Instagram. The predicament of my sort of infertility, is that I'm actually quite fertile. I've never met a pregnancy test I couldn't pass. It's just the making it to a due date that has proven an issue. My eyes crossed as I stumbled upon a language of diagnosis, that I didn't know I would need fluency in. For example, TTC stands for *trying to conceive*. Women would put that acronym in their bios to let potential followers know that they were currently trying. Some would go as far to say *TTC ONLY*.

Meaning, if you were taking a break, or approaching pregnancy from any other route other than top priority, you needn't follow. Medical emojis filled the screen and I was bombarded with unpronounceable drugs and procedures as I searched hashtags like *#miscarriage, #infertility, #pregnancyloss,* and *#lossrecovery*. I spent an entire afternoon feeling seen for the first time ever, and just plain ol' depressed. I dipped my toe in the water and started what would be an anonymous page for a little while.

I noticed that other women would follow and unfollow accounts based on your outlook of infertility. The hopefuls stuck with the encouraging posts and optimistic friends. Posting rainbows and pineapples in their images and ending captions with *#claimingmyblessing*. And the more raw and frustrated women stuck with their own kind, as well. Posting selfies of themselves crying on the toilet and slipping in the phrase *not for weak hearted,* in their captions. I understood both sides, but could not single my identity in one affiliation over another. I was so hopeful towards my healing, and simultaneously incredibly pissed and bitter. I needed both, I could have both, I wanted both.

Just when I was about to give up on positing anything of my own and finding a likeminded friend, I found a profile that kind of looked like mine. Her Instagram handle was simply, *LB*. She only posted minimal images in sepia tones and her captions cut to the chase. She wrote in a way that matched

my emotions of emptiness and being held in numbness. I
followed, liked her only three images, and then I put my
phone down for the evening. The next morning, I laid in bed
for too long scrolling social media, a habit that I hate, but
have no plans to change.

I logged into my new account and saw that *LB* had
celebrated her thirty-fifth birthday the evening before. She
wrote about how she wanted to cancel, but it gave her
something to look forward to, and she kept thinking the
whole night about how she was supposed to be eighteen
weeks pregnant, but she wasn't.

I had nothing to lose, she was anonymous, and I had only
posted my name and just had fifteen followers. With
anonymity on my side, I sent her a message.

Hey. I'm Bailey.

*I just started this page yesterday and I didn't think I would
find so many other pages like mine, but wow. I'm blown
away at the number of women who hurt like me.*

*The post about your birthday touched a part of me that is
still so raw. My husband and I are going through a loss now.
I've been through this a few times before and it only gets
harder.*

I'm here if you ever need to talk.

Best,
B

In her reply, she introduced herself as Lauren. Lauren shared
with me that she had suffered two losses pretty close
together and, to my delight, she was Australian.

In between messages where we discussed our shared hurt
and misfortune, we bonded over an admiration for our stellar
husbands, pasta and homemade pizzas, and a good glass of
wine. She asked me why Americans overuse the words
awesome and *amazing*, while I asked her if she'd ever boxed
a kangaroo, or if she was a good surfer. For a time, Lauren
was my go-to girl. Any feeling of anger or bitterness was
accepted in her grace and if needed, she would match my
emotions and we would throw ourselves a seventeen-hour
delayed pity party. We would share memes and pass along
holistic fertility advice, and songs. When she was getting
ready for her week on Monday morning, I would be having a
lazy Sunday afternoon. The idea that someone I loved and
trusted was already experiencing tomorrow, was an odd
comfort.

One day, Lauren encouraged me to move forward with an
idea that I'd explored a few months earlier. "Have you given
any more thought to starting that group?" I wanted to host a
get-together at my home for women that I knew who were
struggling like me. I could count on both hands the number
of women I knew that experienced loss or couldn't get
pregnant, the battle would be getting them all in one spot
without feeling like we were on a group therapy session.

"I think I'm finally going to do it!" I replied.

I started on my list of names and phone numbers and began
texting the ladies who I thought would want to join my little
club. A club of almost moms. Most of them responded with
a resounding yes. They couldn't wait and asked what they
could bring. A few had to think on it and shared with me

they were still processing their own emotions and didn't
know if a group discussion would be what they needed.

And one responded, "I literally can't think of anything
worse. Thank you, but I'm not interested in coming to that."

Before I knew it, on a Sunday afternoon in August, my home
was filled with really strong and funny women. They were
hopeful and frustrated, brokenhearted and calm. All of us
meeting over our contradicting emotions on the road to
motherhood. We each shared stories of doctors we liked, and
doctors we didn't trust. We shared battle stories and made
lists of stupid things that people say to cheer you up. And we
sat in silence, passing around boxes of Kleenex when we got
to the dark corners of our history. That little group was solid
for a few months. We met a couple of times and encouraged
each other through group text messages.

But as proven of the age-old adage, *nothing keeps*. One by
one, each woman that sat around my dinner table a few
months before, each made their own pregnancy
announcements.

Their ships had come in.

Leaving myself and one other, odd women out.

There is a gross stereotype around women who either can't
get pregnant, or keep pregnancies, or can't produce breast
milk, or can't…whatever. The stereotype is that those
women who are the *have-nots*, are so jealous of the *haves*,
that they will just about strangle them and steal their
children, or bags of colostrum to keep for themselves. I think
this comes from some Disney backfile where soon-to-be

wicked queens stole young wholesome princesses for
themselves or their access to the fountain of youth.

But regular women—the women you work with, or go to
church with, or pass in the grocery store—we are capable of
much more restraint than an evil Disney queen. We can be
so over-the-moon joyful for our friends who get pregnant
while we suffer. We can ache and scream, and still know
that our friends will be wonderful parents. We can still cheer
you on and hurt for ourselves at the same time. Women are
made for so much more than we give ourselves credit for.

From adolescence, we balance the scale of being confident,
but not cocky. Talented, but not too talented to where we
become threats. Beautiful, but not hot. Sexy, but never
slutty. Smart, but not smarter than the boys. Helpful, but not
brownnosers. So, when you worry if the women in your life
will struggle with mustering up joy for someone else who
gets a victory when they are saddled with a loss, don't worry
about them. That will be the one thousandth time they
humbly applauded someone who won the race while they
came in second.

On the heels of my fourth loss, Kyle and I agreed to take a
break from trying. We were tired. I was so done with being
poked and prodded for blood work, and we discovered on
the back end that insurance did not cover a genetic test. And
we were in the hole $5,000.

During that time, my phone rang, and it was my nineteen-
year-old niece. My eldest sister's first born. A petite,
spunky, and beautiful young girl whom I'd adored since she
came barreling into our lives in 2001. She had gone through
some hard times herself in her short years, but she managed
to pull herself up and get into beauty school in Nashville.

Not long after graduating from high school and moving to
Music City, she found a tall fellow who played guitar to run
around town with. And when my phone rang that day, I must
admit, I figured that she needed my help, and we were going
to keep her mother out of it. What I was told instead, was
that she was going to be a mother. To twins.

Breathing, two, one. Exhale, two, one.

There is no punch like the gut punch when the generation
behind you pulls ahead in life steps. If I do say so myself, I
gave an Oscar worthy performance. With my gasps, and
congratulations, and well wishes of, "You will be such a
good mom!" I steadied my voice and didn't allow not one
crack or whimper. I wished her well and told her to call me
if she needed anything. Then I hung up the phone and once
again felt that familiar primal roar bellow from my gut. I
was so stunned that I couldn't form a single sentence to tell
Kyle what happened. Instead, I crawled my way to my
bathtub, filled it up to the brim, and sank down below the
surface to scream underwater.

I did so with such zeal, that I burst a blood vessel in my left
eye.

I knew of nothing else to do, but text my Aussie confidant.
Lauren came through, like she always did. And my timing
couldn't have been worse.

So Bailey,

*I really need to tell you something. And I've put it off
because I didn't know how to do it. Every time I've written
this message, I deleted it because I didn't want to cause you*

*pain, but this has gone on so long I feel like I've betrayed
our friendship by keeping this from you. I'm so sorry about
my timing.*

I'm sorry if I hurt you.

But I'm pregnant.

She was, in fact, almost eight months pregnant. And what
timing it all was. The coronavirus was making landfall in the
United States and her home nation of Australia had been
burning for months. I immediately called her and we both
cried. Joy and sorrow collide when you get what you've
always wanted. Getting what you've always wanted is
terrifying.

I once again felt such joy for a dear friend, and also knew
that I was being left behind. Lauren would be giving birth to
a son, and I knew that she was nervous and elated. We
talked for almost an hour and she promised to send me her
ultrasound images to show me the soft profile of her baby's
face.

When Lauren and I began our friendship over Instagram, we
talked about everything. I knew from the beginning that she
wasn't religious, and she knew that I was a Christian. After
she told me she was pregnant, she sent me a lovely message
encouraging me to take care of myself during this time and
to not lose faith. *Faith.* I'd lost my faith more times than I
could count, and it was soothing to hear someone who
wasn't a believer, mention a belief in something neither of
us could see. I could feel her urgency and support that
almost felt like horsepower through the phone.

"I want this for you so badly, so much so that I imagine this is what a prayer feels like," she told me.

It is a prayer, my love.

That is exactly what prayer feels like.

9

Uncomfortable Comfort and One Less Follower

Here is an uncomfortable truth—our society is populated by people who are not comfortable being uncomfortable. I want to blame the younger generation on social media, or the current obsession with sweatpants, but I think we've always been this way. We don't want to be stuck in conversations we don't like, we don't want to wear pants with zippers, and we don't want to put in the work of facing hard things.

This new wave of self-care has left little room for icky feelings of failure, or grief, or awkwardness amongst our peers. We like neat and tidy people, with neat and tidy posts or messages. And if they've been through anything hard, we don't want to know about it until they are over it. *You better not share your story until you're sure it has a happy ending.* Raw honesty hasn't always been welcomed in some social settings, but honesty is particularly challenging when you can barely face yourself in the mirror for a daily pep-talk during your most uncomfortable days.

You can do this. Come on. You can do it. Just brush your
teeth, run your errands, answer the phone. Then, you can go
back to bed.

It's hard enough to be a human being with your own issues,
but even harder to be there for other human beings and their
issues, too. We aren't comfortable being uncomfortable, and
we also aren't comfortable asking for what we need, which
just leaves relationships bobbing on a buoy of complacency
and barely-there survival. Having a conversation with a
loved one who is ill or depressed, or heartbroken, or rejected
is like drudging through maple syrup. You can walk away,
but you are left sticky from the weight of the conversation,
and then sometimes, if you weren't in the mood to be sticky,
you blame that other person for pulling you through their
sludge of hurt.

A dear friend of mine called me one afternoon a few years
ago. She wanted a baby so badly she couldn't stand it, and
had been trying really hard to start her family for over a
year. Trying so hard in fact, that sex had become a chore,
she monitored her temperature every day, and forbid her
husband to wear boxer-briefs, or use the heated seat feature
in his truck. Something about heated balls wasn't ideal for
sperm quality. *The more you know.*

I had not yet faced any of my own losses. So, I assumed, as
most folks do, that she was being dramatic, and that she was
rushing her life. She threw around the word *infertility,* and I
laughed at her and said, "You're being too hard on yourself!
Just have a glass of wine and let the magic happen when it
happens. Throw out that thermometer, girl!" What an
insensitive bitch I was. I didn't know what I didn't know.
And even in my ignorance, I didn't want to be pulled into
her uncomfortable truth.

There has to be space for both. I think the world is big
enough and we are complex enough to exist in a place where
you can do your self-care routine, honor self-preservation,
and still be available to sit next to your friend who is
devastated that life is not turning out the way she thought it
would. There can be a common place of existence where you
can give her a bag of lavender infused Epsom salts, and tell
her to go take a bath, while you fold her clothes, and brush
her hair that's been tangled from living in a bed of
depression for four months. Or at the very least, we should
be able to sit through a phone call and listen to a friend use
words we hate to hear, words like infertility.

Self-care isn't the end all be all goal, self-care is an assisted
means of survival. It's the guardrail you run into while you
shake off life's latest hit and look around to make sure
everyone else is okay, too.

I figured all this out the hard way when people would ask,
"Hey, how are you holding up?" when I would see them in
the grocery store or out-and-about after my losses. I would
give an honest answer, like I always have, and then I would
realize that my real response was not what they were looking
for.

They were just being polite and making small talk.

Small talk doesn't involve real responses.

I would slowly read the regret and terror in their eyes, and
discover they didn't want to know the answer to whatever
question they'd just asked. My real answer is uncomfortable,
my real answer holds emotion, and my real answer will
sound like regret, and grief, and embarrassment.

My real answer will have nothing to do with the weather, or surface level banter, and everything to do with existing in a world that I've questioned to live in.

After my sister lost her child, people eventually stopped asking me how she was doing. Because I would tell them the truth. "She left work early today and went home to lay in her daughter's bed." *Oh.* They didn't want to know that. They just wanted me to say, "She is okay and doing as expected. Thanks for asking."

I don't know of any other way to be. I have no time to mince words. I have no time to be fake. I have no time to filter my answers for other people's comfort level. I prefer getting down to brass tacks and standing in my truth. And my truth sometimes looks like depression. It sometimes looks like failure. It sometimes looks like rage. It sometimes looks like a great peace and contentment that catches me off guard. And, on very rare occasions, it will look like a scene from a *Nancy Meyers* film, in which case, I post that shit on Instagram ayy-sap.

I share the grey parts, too.

I won't say too much about the time of my niece's death, the story is not mine to tell. But I can say this—the people who stick around long enough to ask how your family is doing and sit with you as you ugly cry over the unspeakable loss of a precious child—those are my people. The people who never mention it ever again and brush over the topic and pretend it didn't happen, those are *not* my people.

I know it's uncomfortable, so was junior high.

I just grew so tired of it. I'm so tired of women feeling like they have to be better than what they are. How you are, is perfect, even in your smelly sweatpants that you've worn every day for a month. For the first few years after we were married, I struggled to find women that I could relate to. I was surrounded by women who loved their jobs, had stair-step kids fourteen months apart, they worked, but they didn't have to, and they never seemed to have zits or issues. They all dressed the same, drove the same SUV, carried the same purse, and wore the same perfume. I couldn't recognize myself in those women. I didn't feel welcomed in those circles.

I needed women around me who rolled their eyes at the over filtered, blush toned squares on their Instagram feed, too. Everything is not perfect. And that is where I want to be, the unperfect place.

Give me the women who are barely hanging on. Give me the women who have found a way to laugh at their own instability. Give me the women who are fighting tooth and nail, who are white knuckling it through their days and somehow still have enough left over to give their children, community, and their friends. Give me the women who forget to wear perfume and use the same purse they've carried since college. I want to sit at a crowded table with women who lay out the honesty of their shortcomings and anger, their frustrations and celebrations, their weight gain and mental health. Give me those women.

I got so sick of being surrounded by women who perpetuate the idea that life is always Instagramable and never broken. Never tired. Never angry. Never uncomfortable.

After my first two miscarriages, I shared some of my more raw moments in an effort to not feel so alone. Shortly after, I received a message on Instagram from someone who wanted to politely inform me, that she was unfollowing me.

_____

Hey Bailey,

I've enjoyed following your posts over the last few years, but I think I'm going to have to unfollow you for a bit. Lately you've really just been posting heavy and sad stuff. And I think you have such a positive voice that you aren't using. Maybe you should try to focus on the good and not the bad for a change? People don't want to be depressed when they are on social media. This isn't really the place for that.

Good luck, girl!

_____

I never responded to her. I was too stunned and embarrassed. But I did become quite paranoid for a while that people viewed me as sad, and only sad. As if my few, very open and honest posts about real life was the only quality left to my name. I developed a fear that when people heard my name or thought of me, they pictured a snotty, red-faced woman who couldn't get out of bed. Now I wonder what that woman was facing on her own. Why couldn't she stand to see my hurt on her feed? I've wondered if it was because her hurt got in the way of her observing mine, too.

But the thing is…I'm not sad. Not all the time. And even if I was, I can't care if it makes you uncomfortable. My temporary sadness can exist independently of my person.

And so could hers.

Sad things have happened to me. Sad things have happened around me. I guess you could say I'm sad adjacent. But just because heartache chose to follow me around for the last six years doesn't mean that I, myself, am *only* sad. I'm much more than my temporary emotions.

You are so much more than your temporary emotions.

People are entitled to feel shitty over the way that life has burned them. That's the fun part of being a human. The magical rendering to all of it, is this: most of the people you know, even the happiest and prettiest, most well put together people, have crushing tales of their own. And I firmly believe most of them *want* to share those stories. We don't have to live in a bad Zoloft commercial forever, but we can at least hunker down to hear the hard stuff, to share the hard stuff.

A few summers ago, my dear friend, Taylor, told me that she was expecting her first child. She'd lost her mother to pancreatic cancer the previous winter, and I know she was overjoyed to extend the love her mother left behind down to her own son.

The waters of our friendship became murky due to bad timing and big feelings. The rough edges of life scraped us as we poorly navigated her grief and pregnancy, alongside my fourth loss. For a short time in the month of June, we were pregnant at the same time. Just as she was revealing the gender of her firstborn, I was lying in my bed and could feel my insides pull and burn as the sac detached from my uterine wall. I sent her a brief text message updating her on the loss. And she responded a few days later, with a sonogram picture of her son.

Big feelings.

Bad timing.

A strained friendship ensued.

I couldn't have known how desperately she wanted to send
the sonogram image to her mother. She needed me to share
in her joy, and I couldn't. She didn't understand that I
couldn't bear to look at a staticky picture of her baby. I
needed a friend. She needed a friend to take the place of her
mom. Two women were lost in the stickiness of hurt, unable
to pull from the grips. We were uncomfortable and at a dead
end. Not knowing any better and not having the emotional
capacity to fix it, I drew a self-care boundary line in the sand
and told her not to cross it.

She felt rejected and overlooked. I felt mocked and bruised,
as if she'd kicked me while I was down. Uncomfortability
sucked the air out of an eight-year friendship.

At the time, I didn't know I could do both. I didn't know that
I could lay down a boundary and not walk away entirely. I
don't think Taylor knew that I could hold congratulations for
her and not be an active participant in the day-to-day
growing's at the same time. My joy for her could exist
independently from the sorrow that I held for me. We didn't
know that we could've loved, and supported each other from
a healthy distance, and not risked getting stuck in the
thorned weeds of heartache. It took time, but we know now.

Taylor reached out to me after her son was born. She said
the thought of never being able to hold him made her think
of me. She apologized for sending sonogram pictures and
sounds of his heartbeat at such a delicate time. And I

apologized for having been all or nothing in my support, especially the nothing.

I know better now about my boundaries. I observe them and take note of them. I file them behind limits, pet peeves, and personal quirks. Which include but are not limited to:

House covered in dog hair.

Weird smells.

People being rude to waitstaff.

People who are habitually late.

Overextending myself to prove my worth to others.

Eating artichokes straight from the jar.

People responding to a text with just 'K.'

Not voicing my needs in a quick effort to survive complacency.

People are uncomfortable around me when I reveal that I know about *baby stuff*. Their eyes widen in confusion when I ask if the baby is sleeping through the night, or if they have a good latch, do they have cradle cap, or jaundice. They are physically uncomfortable telling me they have mastitis, and that their baby won't sleep longer than fifteen minutes. I know about baby stuff. It comes with the territory of infertility and having friends who are all parents.

A friend once asked me what all this is like. She wanted to know what infertility felt like, and I'm so glad she didn't feel uncomfortable asking me. The best way I can describe it, is comparing it to winning the lottery.

You won!

You got the check!

You've made arrangements to pay off all your debt, you bought your dream home, and just as you're about to retire and change your whole life, they take it back. There was a mistake, a miscalculation, the wrong number was called. The winnings are not yours to keep. You only got a glimpse of what your life could look like and just as you fell in love with a future you wouldn't know—they take it all back. The stretching and shrinking is what hurts the most. The stretching to a future you're desperately trying to grasp, and then forcing yourself to shrink back to the way you were before, never exactly fitting the same ever again.

I'm very cozy laying in a pallet of uncomfortableness now. I've made a grief fort and waited for the phone to ring for others to join me in there, and I was surprised to find out so few of my loved ones called to check-in. The strained place of growing and stretching in uncomfortableness hurt. Growing pains usually do.

It hurts in the weirdest and best way.

I've covered myself with weighted blankets of big uncomfortable feelings, and let fate do her work while I rest. I like that place. That icky, stretching, restful, uncomfortable place—it's where I've grown the most.

10

Thanks for Being an F'ing Friend

My mother bestowed lots of pieces of advice upon me during my formative years. In particular, she had a never-ending list of tips on how to gain friends. Looking back now, I think she was just trying to get me to do things that I didn't want to do, and she was preparing me for my interesting tour in therapy, but the advice is still pretty solid.

You better go brush your teeth! No one wants to have a friend with rot-mouth.

Go take a bath! No one wants to be friends with a smelly Sally!

You better stop with that attitude! Nobody wants to be friends with a diva!

You better be nice to people, no one will hang out with a sourpuss.

*Learn how to be a good loser, if you're a poor sport, no one
will want to play with you.*

*Never talk about yourself too much, no one wants to talk
about you all the time.*

You have to be a friend, in order to have friends.

Besides giving me an obsessive phobia about smelling bad,
the advice was well received. Friendships can be odd and
tricky relationships that I don't think we invest enough time
into tending. You grow what you water, and I'm not sure
people have green thumbs when it comes friendships
nowadays.

In college, I met a beautiful friend named Hardy. She
casually mentioned that not every friend is supposed to be
your best friend, and as someone who's spent her entire life
searching for a deep connection with every single person
I've come in to contact with, that was an explosion of
freedom for me. She was right. Not every person who you
consider a friend, will be your best friend.

I've been told the friends you keep, either have a big *F* or a
little *f*.

And this is how you categorize your f'ing friends.

I have a theory that you need both F's in different ways. The
big *F* friends are the people who help you plan your mom's
funeral. They help you pack up your home during a divorce.
They sit with you on the floor after heartache, until you're
ready to stand up again. They take you on trips to get you
out of town when you need a breather. They run to the
grocery store for you. They know where you hide the good

liquor in the back of your cabinets. They loan you money with zero expectations of you paying them back.

The big *F* friends hold enough confidence that you don't have to talk every day, but they are a constant for you.

One of my oldest F'ing friends is Haley. My beautiful Haley Jo. She sat behind me in second grade, and she was so painfully shy that I would have to order her lunch for her in the cafeteria line. She, like many others, usually never knows what to say to me when hard days come. But when my phone lights up with her face and name on the screen, it's enough. Hearing her voice and childlike laughter is like going home for me. She is known for obsessing over weather updates and is adorably manic when storms come to town. She is one of the few people that I can peacefully travel with, and her fear of heights matches my own. Haley has sat on the phone with me for more hours than I can count. She and I have the same affinity for a clean kitchen, and she is a really good soul. She is one of my favorite big F'ing friends.

The little f'ing friends are the same treasures, just in different ways. Those are the friends you occasionally have lunch with, and you can bounce career ideas off of them. They may have a child in the same grade as yours and you can text about being annoyed with science fair criteria. They are really supportive on your social media feeds and they remember to ask how your spouse is doing, too.

A rarity, a lovely surprise to fill your days, is when the little *f* friends, become the big *F* friends. I met Sarah through a mutual friend about eight years ago. She is blonde and beautiful, thoughtful with her prayers and you'd never guess it, but she is a Kung-Fu instructor. Her tiny little frame can break your wrists before you even realize it. I can't exactly remember when Sarah moved from the lower-case *f*, to the capital grade *F*, but she was the only person who stood in the muck of my fourth miscarriage with me. She wasn't afraid to go to the dark places and she never shied away from tough conversations. She texted me scriptures and encouragement the morning of my surgery, and her texts haven't stopped since. She spoke words over me that I desperately needed to hear. She is the type of woman who shows up for you, time and time again. She is a good F'ing friend.

Not long after Kyle and I started dating, we took a day trip from Starkville, Mississippi down to Jackson. We met up with one of my old college roommates and spent the day shopping and dining. We enjoyed a sushi lunch, and I was amazed that I actually liked yellowtail. After eating way too many edamame, we began walking around a gorgeous outdoor shopping center. Having grown up in a very small town, the closest shopping was about a forty-minute drive away, and it was just your average mall.

The one we strolled that day had marble fountains, an *Apple* store, *Sephora*, and a fairly new *Anthropologie*. Marissa, my friend from college, had taken a summer job at that *Anthropologie* a few years back and still knew most of the staff. She and I walked in and marveled at the candles and jewelry, eclectic bedding, and houseware. We caught up on life as we ran our fingers over their dresses that we didn't have the confidence or money to buy.

I was looking at a lime green sheep fur pullover that cost $259 when the yellowtail and edamame I'd enjoyed earlier, forcefully informed me they were ready to make their exit. My stomach began expanding and shrinking like an accordion and sweat started to run down my spine. This was quickly becoming a pressing issue.

I calmly walked over to Marissa and asked where the
restroom was. She told me they didn't have a restroom open
to the public, but she knew the manager was cool and would
let me run in really fast.

What happened next was a blur. My restroom visit turned
into a war zone in under five minutes. I will spare you the
details and just say the white lie that I told the manager, *it's
just number one,* was about to haunt me for years to come. It
in fact, was not just number one. I gave that toilet a good
talking-to and then tried to flush with no luck. I jiggled the
nob and tried to flush again. Water was rising quickly. Like,
Titanic-level, Jack-and-Rose-running-down-the-hallway,
rising quickly. Ingenuity kicked in, and I quickly leaned
down behind the toilet to turn the water off. Just before it
began to run down the sides of the commode.

I was stuck. There was no plunger. There was no way out.
How the hell was I going to explain this to my friend and her
former boss? I was in a store that sold eighty-dollar
potholders, and I'd just destroyed their plumbing. The water
taunted me as it bobbed back and forth, skimming the edge,
but never falling over, and by then I was in a full-blown
sweat meltdown.

I'm not proud of what I did next, but I felt it was my only
option.

I washed my hands, straightened my shirt, and turned to the
pastel yellow, shabby chic shelf that stood next to the sink. I
then proceeded to unroll an entire spool of heavy-duty
Bounty paper towels and shoved them in the toilet.

I had to make a run for it at some point. And this was the
only way I could see me opening the door and hauling ass. I

pushed that last square of paper towels in the bowl, turned off the light, and ran like hell. I found Marissa over by the hand-dipped candles and said, "We have to get out of here immediately." I called Kyle and told him that I had a headache and was ready to leave. Both he and Marissa stared at me in confusion as I behaved like a crazed felon who had just escaped from prison.

The next day I got a phone call from Marissa. She'd heard from an old coworker at *Anthropologie* who'd reached out to say that it was good to see her. Before the end of their text conversation, her former coworker said, "And don't worry. I cleaned up the mess, and I won't tell anyone."

"Bails, what did you do? He said something about a clogged toilet?"

I confessed right there. I had nowhere to hide, and I was fresh out of paper towels. We laughed at the bathroom debacle and Marissa said, "Well he thought I was the one who did it and I didn't correct him, so you're good to go back in there. They don't have your mugshot in the breakroom or anything."

I'm not sure what *F* category that falls under, but that is a good fucking friend.

To this day, I've not stepped foot back into an *Anthropologie*.

Six months before we were married, Kyle and I went to a couple's seminar at church. The keynote speakers were two married psychologists who wrote self-help books about their love, faith, and fighting fairly. We never attended pre-marital counseling, so we figured at the very least, watching another married couple air their dirty laundry on stage could be helpful. We took our seats, and I turned around to spy two familiar faces. I'd just taken a new job, and I saw my coworker and his wife sitting right behind us. I'm not sure why I got so excited. I barely knew them, but the idea of seeing a couple our age outside of work was a needed glimpse of routine. Kyle and I had recently moved to the Jackson area and we had no friends to call for dinner, or coffee, or to have over to watch a football game.

My eyes lit up at their familiar faces and to my husband's surprise, I asked them to join us for dinner after the seminar. They politely agreed, and I can't explain what their *yes* meant to me. I took it as the first building block to establish our community in a new town. The seminar was over two hours long, so halfway through, we paused for a bathroom break. I ran into the wife in the restroom, and I made small talk. She confirmed that they were starving, too. I can't remember what tipped me off, but something about how she looked me up and down, gave me a red flag that she was very suspicious of me.

I once again pushed for the dinner confirmation and she echoed a yes, but wasn't as enthusiastic as before. As the seminar came to a close, I bent down to collect our newly-signed marriage advice books and turned to say we would see them at the restaurant.

What we saw instead, was the back of their heads as the wife briskly pushed her husband away from us and towards the door. She peaked over her shoulder to see if we saw her, and I can only assume I looked like a stunned loser, with a capital *L*.

I came on too strong. No one tells you how to make friends in your twenties. Maybe I should've just asked for their

number before asking them out? But it was in that moment
that I prayed for that couple. I prayed they would never
know a day where they so desperately needed a friend as
much as we did that night.

I felt so foolish, but over time I've realized how gaining and
maintaining friendships as an adult is *never* discussed. *Ever.*
No one told me that moving to a new town would be so
difficult. Nobody told me that people my age weren't
currently taking applications for new friends, or well-paying
jobs for that matter. Not a soul warned me that nurturing
friendships as you get older is like a part-time job.

Friends aren't always going to say the right things, they
aren't always going to understand your humor, they
definitely aren't always going to take the blame for your
bathroom catastrophes, and they may sometimes forget your
birthday. But the good friends are worth the wait. The good
friends won't walk out when you need them most. The value
of a good friend, lower case or capital *F*, will always be
worth tending to. I'm blessed with lots of f'ing friends
today, but that took years of eating lunch alone and learning
to be kind to myself in the meantime.

Mama at least got one piece of advice right. You have to be
a friend, in order to have friends.

11

Catch And Release

My dad is a *catch and release* kind of fisherman. He doesn't
fish for food or sport, it's only a leisurely pastime he enjoys
in his golden years. He is a patient man who will sit on his
dock for hours, just waiting for a nibble. When he reels one
in, he will examine their gills and scales, take a picture to
text me or my mom, and then gently unhook them to place
back in the lake. I find his philosophy of catching and
releasing bass quite reflective of his own personality. The
man's personal motto is, *it's all good.*

When I was very small, my dad would pick me up from
school every Friday and drive with the windows down as
Hootie & the Blowfish sang us home. The unmistakable
stench of New Orleans would whisk into the car as we made
our way from downtown to the Westbank, and even as a
young child, I knew the air felt different on Friday
afternoons. My dad is a Tennessee native who taught me
from a young age to never tolerate bullying. He, himself,
was the victim of such cruelty during his formative years
and it shaped, or rather, misshaped who he is today.

He would say things like, "Don't ever make someone feel beneath you." Or "Putting people down to make you feel taller is not who we are." He is the epitome of one who never judges a book by their cover. And when shaking hands, my father would always offer his grip palm facing up, instead of down. I wouldn't learn until my senior year of college in a course that studied body language, that this was a sign of not only respect, but a docile gesture. He gladly handed over control and authority to other people if he felt like they needed it more.

One of my first memories is of him escorting an elderly lady and her walker, across a busy street. The sweetness in him is something that I pray to inherit. A true gentleman, he is good and humble. Kind and hard working. Honest and wanting. But even the kindest of us, have our breaking points.

When I was growing up, he would surprise me with donuts after school, and dance with my mother around the kitchen, but he was also known to over work until the point of exhaustion, leaving little of himself left over for his marriage or children. My father is the kind of man who, when our hometown church split because of business decisions, he offered our front lawn as a place to worship until we found a new building, and he had a cross built for the new sanctuary long before we knew where it would stand. I was around thirteen when I learned the bully he was so often at the mercy of in his childhood, was his own father. A generation of meanness and abuse was alive and well inside his memories.

After you learn that someone you love was hurt as a child, if you stare at him long enough, the broken boy inside of him will appear right before your eyes.

It's a lot easier to take your time molding and raising children than it is to heal broken adults.

I'm not sure if it was the pressure of responsibilities, my mother having cancer twice in a four-year span, unhealed childhood trauma, or maybe his life just wasn't turning out the way he had planned; but, around the time that I started middle school, he began to slip in and out of spells of depression and sobriety. Depression wasn't discussed in the nineties and early two-thousands. And if it was discussed, it sure wasn't talked about by middle-aged men in south Mississippi. I can remember watching him come home after work, the man was utterly exhausted and unsure of himself. I wish so badly I could go back in time and pull on the hem of my mother's skirt and say, "Pay attention. This is where we lose him."

The days blended together in a salty-sweet flow from my own adolescence to young adulthood, and before I knew it, for no particular reason—but rather several reasons I couldn't name—I myself, was slipping in and out of depression and panic.

I was in my sophomore year at Mississippi State University. I had changed my major for the fourth time, and my GPA reflected such decisions of a finicky nineteen-year-old. I had no idea what I wanted to do with my life, and I didn't feel like I belonged anywhere amongst my friends or classmates. Gap years should really be more accepted in our culture.

To observe a group of college students is really like watching a drunken circus. There are cliques of young people who are balancing the tight rope of independence and confusion, while they cling to the juvenility from which they ran so quickly to escape from. They are forced to juggle the idea of adulthood, when they've never felt more like a child.

Everyone becomes an arm-chair psychologist after holding their roommate's hair back during the first football weekend, or having a tipsy heart-to-heart in a bathroom stall, and every single one of them is looking for love in all the wrong places.

Whooo. What a precious time. What a shit-show.

I was an active participant in that circus when my father was diagnosed with a laundry list of health issues that forced him into early retirement. I quickly discovered that life doesn't stop throwing curve balls at you just because you're trying to earn a higher education.

We were approaching the deadline in the semester where you either stuck it out or dropped for the year. I was sitting in a small classroom as my professor started naming projects and their due dates, along with extra credit and internship opportunities. I was taking notes and trying not to think about my dad lying in a hospital bed three-hundred miles away, when an odd squeal started to echo from somewhere in the classroom. When my teacher turned to me with a panicked look, I realized the squeal was coming from me. I was trying to breathe, but as air got trapped in the back of my throat, that natural task seemed to be proving a challenge.

I was having my first panic attack.

In class.

In front of my professor and peers.

Yay!

*Step right up, folks! Here is your chance to see a young lady
who has taken a big bite out of life and is struggling like a
fish out of water! Up next, financial-aid flame throwers!*

My embarrassing squeal only got louder in my efforts to
hush myself, and I couldn't decide which to be embarrassed
about first. The fact that I was showing weakness and failure
in a crowded room, or the fact that my weakness and failure
sounded like a strangled cat.

Decisions, decisions.

In a heroic and poised move, my professor calmly asked all
other students to excuse themselves and she sat in front of
me telling me that I was okay. She repeated the words,
"You're okay. You're safe. Just breathe," until I started to
believe her. She even drove me to the student health-plex
and waited for me to be checked out by a nurse who
informed me that I'd suffered a panic attack.

I'd never heard of them until that moment.

After I regulated my breathing, I walked across the Drill
Field and found myself sitting on the concrete steps of Lee
Hall. It was a beautiful spring afternoon. The sun was hiding
behind McCool Hall allowing for the most gorgeous orange-
sherbet glow to fall over campus. The dogwood trees were
regaining their blooms and other students that passed by me
would smile or say hello, and I had to reteach myself how to
respond with smiles and waves after such an experience. I
watched other students and faculty walk from one end of
campus to the other, no one else seemed to be struggling. No
one else looked as if they were failing. No one else's eyes
were bloodshot with stress and humiliation. But they had to
be, right? I couldn't be the only one who was overwhelmed
with the idea of a future that I wasn't ready for but seemed

to be barreling towards me at the speed of light. Looking back, I wonder what the rush was? There is nothing special about working and paying taxes, but there is something extraordinarily special about finding your place and slowly understanding who you are to yourself.

For the first time ever, I was approaching a place of freedom that I would learn to welcome in my life.

The freedom of doing nothing.

Over the years, my mother has been full of advice, solicited and otherwise. Most of her advice is fantastic, and her other nuggets of wisdom could get us kicked out of church. But one of her tried and true, go-to pieces of life-lessons is this: *When you don't know what to do, do nothing.* I didn't know what to do, so it seemed that my only choice was to do nothing at all.

Internships and exams, my dad living long enough to leave the hospital, strained friendships, chapter meetings, swap-dates, passed due rent, learning to stand on my own two feet, and all the other horribly exciting and daunting things that new adults face—it was all staring at me, watching me fail and waiting for me to respond. And the only thing I knew to do, the only response that I knew to hand over, was to eliminate the things I had control over (which wasn't much) and leave the things that I had no control over (like my dad living or dying) to sort themselves out.

I stood from the cold steps of Lee Hall and walked straight to the Dean's office to drop-out for the semester. I focused on working until I understood what I really wanted to do with my life, or at least until I narrowed in on a major that could help me get there.

While I was in the Dean's office, I met an angel of a woman
named Barbara Stewart. Barbara will hold a dear place in my
heart as long as I live. I didn't know this beforehand or else I
would've prepared a speech, but you need a reason to drop
out. A formal reason that will go on your record of why you
feel that you can't complete the school year. I sobbed in
front of poor Barbara's desk, trying to pick just one reason
for her to type into the computer, and she gently handed me
a tissue from her maroon shelf. In between my cries that
once again felt like a panic attack, I explained that it was all
too much. My dad's declining health, I'd just been dumped,
study hall, and partying, exams, and volunteer hours, friends
who never seemed to get me, my foreign language professor
insisted on speaking only in French for the duration of class
and French turned out to be way harder than I thought, and
not near as romantic. A lot of spit sounds are involved. I
couldn't find my way. I didn't feel like me. How was I ever
supposed to find my way in this world when I couldn't
manage to stop crying long enough to explain that I was lost.

Barbara Stewart handed me one more Kleenex, slowly
turned her chair to face me, and then proceeded to give me
the most profound advice I would ever hear.

"That is a lot to handle right now. Have you thought about
speaking with a therapist?"

A therapist?

No ma'am.

The thought never occurred to me. Mrs. Stewart was the first
person in my life who would ever encourage me to take care
of my mental health. She was the first person to give me
permission to take a break and regroup so I could be better.

Her kindness that day changed my life, if not saved it
entirely.

I wondered why my father had never come across a Barbara
Stewart of his own. How different his life could've been if
just one person had told him to take a breather.

After I left the Dean's office, I withdrew my pin from my
sorority, dropped out of the handful of clubs I was in, and
put my stressed-out ass in therapy. It was quite the
Thursday.

Shortly after that pivotal day, I heard my dad's voice for the
first time in two weeks. He was conscious, alert, and
preparing to leave the hospital.

"Hey, Peanut."

I sobbed when I heard his scratchy mumble. The weight of
the world was lifted and even if it was just for one more day,
I got to keep my dad. He tried as best as he could to make
small talk and ask me about school, and my sorority, and my
friends. I swallowed my pride and told him I had, well, I had
nothing to update him on, because I currently held nothing
but a job at a local pre-school.

"I'm going to take some time off school and refocus. This
will give me more time to come visit you an—" The words
were still rolling their way from my mouth to the phone
when he stopped me.

"Good heavens, girl. No! You will lose your spot and you
will fall behind. Please don't do this because of me."

It took a bit of convincing him and my mom that I was okay, and I promised them I would enroll again in the fall. I needed the break, the respite, the time off from the merry-go-round that was making me sick with anxiety. I swore to them that I would do my best next semester, and I would just take it slow. I think he was still a little loopy from the drugs the hospital had given him because he laughed and said, "Yea, sure. Famous. Last. Words."

We are all entitled to our boundaries and limits, and we need to know where to draw the line in the sand when we've met them. Having a breakdown in public that lead me to feel like a zoo animal was the first of many boundaries I would lay down. I've since learned that my limit for stress and multitasking seems to be a great deal lower than those around me, and that is okay. I've also learned that you only get so many chances to use your voice before you lose it, it's best to speak your mind the first chance you get, especially if it involves your own health and needs. The sun still sets a bit deeper in Starkville, Mississippi, and I was fortunate enough to see that same orange-sherbet glow sweep over campus many more times before I received my diploma.

There comes a time in your life where you face your first huge loss. The foundation of all you know is cracked and the rubble will never allow you to walk the same path again. For me, that was the season when I discovered that my path will never look like the people standing next to me. What a harsh lesson to learn at a young age when all you want to do is look like those standing beside you. I wouldn't fully accept this lesson until I was in my late twenties.

Nothing lasts forever, it's not built to. Even the bad days, the panic attack days, the critical moments that you swear will break you in half; they end too. The best we can do, is when the good shows up, welcome it and enjoy that sweet spot of

all being in its place, relish in it, because that will end, too.
And when the wind changes, as it always will, the only thing
to do is take a deep breath, take note of what you've got, and
what you should let go of—then release.

12

My Mama and Carol King

My mother has no idea that she is beautiful. It's not like she has never been told, she just doesn't believe people when they tell her. What she does know for sure, is that she is wild and insecure, fearless and timid, content and unsettled. Her personality is just as chaotic as her curly hair, and she is known to burst into song when she hears a word that reminds her of a lyric, and she is usually the first person on the dance floor at a wedding. When I was growing up, she would wake me up each morning in a very specific way that was humiliating to me, even though no one else was around. Don't you remember that teenagers can blush with shame in an empty room?

My mama would wake me up by singing and dancing. She would jump on my bed or holler up the stairs and say, "Today is gonna be a ggrrreeaaattttt day!"

And I would hate it.

She would startle me awake by singing *Carol King* or *Janis Joplin* and shake me until I got up with only six minutes to spare before I was late for school. But after I grumbled down

the stairs and refused to meet her level of excitement for the
morning, she would take my hand, open it, and kiss the
center of my palm. Then she would fold my hand back
tightly, and tell me, "My love is in there all day, just in case
you need it." She must have been terrified to face cancer at
only thirty-six years old, but I don't remember her showing
anything but bravery. She showed strength and carried the
air that she simply didn't have time to die. She hid me from
the rough parts of her treatments, and she enjoyed not having
to shave her legs for a while, the only perk of losing all your
hair. I only recently learned over dinner at her sixtieth
birthday, that she was frozen in a kind of fear that only
comes with facing your own death. And I felt I owed her a
great deal when she told me that she fought the way she did,
for me.

"I wasn't going to leave my baby. I will die one day, but I
wasn't going to leave my seven-year-old, and I wasn't going
out of here from cancer. I made sure of that."

*But how did you make sure of it, Mama? We have no control
over these things.*

My mother comes from the generation of hard work and no
room for down time or sadness. The 1960's were fantastic
for so many reasons, particularly the music, but they missed
the mark on mental health. *Hello, Vietnam.* I don't recall her
ever sitting down when I was a kid. She was always on the
move, cleaning or fixing, or sprucing, and the woman never
ate fast food until I was in college. She worked so she
wouldn't have to focus on her insecurities, she persevered so
she could make sure things were done to her standards. She
painted so she could say what she needed to say with oil-
soaked brushstrokes.

I had every intention of hiding my second pregnancy from her until I was in my second trimester, but when you're so used to telling your mom everything, even about your very specific bathroom visits, it's really difficult to keep things like having a child hidden from her. I'd had one miscarriage, and I just knew there was no way that could happen to me again. So when I went to visit my parents one weekend, without my husband, I just about burst into her front door to tell her the good news. I sat on the sofa next to her to cuddle up for a rainy afternoon movie, and I slowly turned to her and whispered, "I'm pregnant, Mama." And then, as it always happens, even though you swear you won't get your hopes up, you make plans.

My overjoyed mother started asking me about names and pre-schools, Christening gowns and nursery color schemes. I walked with her through the daydreams of gender-neutral rooms and which family names we liked best. We told my dad, and we all had a good cry, again being so sure, that this was it, this one would stick. My parents placed bets on whether it was a boy or a girl, and I knew in my bones my Daddy was right, I felt like it was a girl, too. The weekend continued with normalcy, pockets of joy, and random spurts of, "Hey! When you're ready to paint the nursery, you know we will come help." Or "What school district are y'all in?"

We were getting ready for dinner. My dad was cooking in the kitchen and my mom was setting the table. I went to use the restroom. And then…it's just gone. No need to pick names just yet. That spare room will remain spare. Don't worry with schools, you don't need them.

Your stroll through daydreams of a future evaporates in a breathless scream. I can't remember how I got from the bathroom to the couch, or if I called Kyle or my mom did. But all I can remember is the weight of my dad's hand on

my back, and my mom's inaudible whispers as they prayed
over their child, who was losing her child. Without knowing
of anything else to do, my mother clung to any shred of
positivity that she could. "Spotting is normal, honey." She
reminded me of my cousin's wife who had severe bleeding
in the first trimester of each of her pregnancies, and
everything turned out fine.

As any strong spiritual woman does, my mother had holy oil
in her bathroom cabinet. She gave me the bottle to hold after
she put a few drops in her hand and she gently placed her
palm over my stomach. It was a comfort. It provided a peace
that wasn't there minutes before. But it cured nothing. None
of us ate dinner that night. I went to bed early, and woke
several times in the night to pray, and beg that little nugget
to stay put for as long as she could.

By the time the sun rose, the bottle of oil was empty, and so
was I.

For a long time, due to no other reason than us allowing it to
happen, my infertility drove a wedge between me and my
mom. She couldn't understand that her positivity unfolded a
blanket of false hope that I couldn't bear to rest on. And I
couldn't understand that she didn't understand me. For the
first time in my life, my own mother treated me like all the
other people who'd hidden from me, and she simply said
nothing at all. She figured saying nothing was better than
saying the wrong thing.

So, silence did what silence does best, it built a wall between
a parent and child, and neither one of us had the strength to
tear it down.

If you're among the lucky, after a certain age, your parents become your friends. I consider myself one of the lucky. My mother and I have a wonderful friendship beyond our blood.

Which made the wall built by silence all the more painful.

My mom didn't know what to say to me, my friend didn't know what to say to me. She had a faith for me that I couldn't hold on to. She can so easily close her eyes, and picture me pregnant or being a mother, and I just can't anymore. She used the same spitfire spirit to will me into motherhood, that she willed herself into remission. *But how do you know, Mama? We aren't promised such things.*

I've had to remind her over the years that not everyone is as brave as she is, but she doesn't consider herself brave, so this causes confusion. She will be dumbfounded that other people don't make decisions the way she does. For example, when I was in college, I refused to find a new gynecologist in north Mississippi, instead I would rather make the four-hour drive home to see the doctor that I was comfortable with in Louisiana. The problem was, I never took the time to schedule the appointment and the drive. I was cleaning my apartment one Saturday when I was on the phone with her, explaining that I felt a real connection (whatever that means) with that particular doctor, and I knew she didn't judge me, and I don't want to start over with someone new. My mother sharply responded with a one-liner I will carry with me forever.

"Bailey Elizabeth, get over yourself, it's just a pussy."

Yes ma'am.

Before I went to Mississippi State University, I made a short detour through community college. It was the best kind of fun I've ever had, and I guess I got some sort of schooling there, but I really can't remember much about classrooms from that time. My mother drove me to campus and helped me register. And as things like that go, the day was long, and the lines were longer. I had just received my official schedule when realized that I hadn't seen my mother for about an hour. When I called her, she matter-of-factly told me that she was in the cafeteria having lunch—with the entire *Pearl River Community College* football team. If there ever was a time to shit myself, that was it. I walked into the cafeteria with my heart racing in my throat, and I scanned the room for my mother, who was sitting at a table with the entire defensive line. She called me over to introduce me to her new friends, and I shook my head in refusal. She stood from the table and a lovely gentleman who clocked in at six foot six said, "Bye Ms. D, Thanks for the talk." God love her.

It always amazes me that the human brain can trick you or distort your memories. I attended a small Baptist private school in New Orleans, and I had a few lines in a kindergarten play. I remember being so nervous to step up to the short microphone. I know the room was packed. I know moms and dads, aunts and uncles, and teachers filled the seats. But all I can remember is my mom sitting on the empty front row, waving and smiling to me. All I can see, all my memory can hold, is her.

I was lying in the hospital bed waiting for the nurses to roll me back for my D&C during my fourth miscarriage, when I could feel her presence in the room. I could smell her perfume as she came up behind me. She didn't say a word, she didn't know which words to speak. But my mother once again held onto a bottle of holy oil and began calling on the hallways of heaven for her baby. She kissed my forehead at

least thirty times before they rolled me back, and she kissed
my left palm, for good love and luck. And when I woke up,
she was right by my side, holding my hand. She picked up
lunch for me on the way back to my house, and she sat with
me for the rest of the afternoon, mostly in silence.

My mother is still one of my closest friends. It took a while
for us to tear down the wall that silence built. Conversations
of loss are still uncomfortable for us. She is instantly timid,
and I'm already on the defense when the topic turns to IVF
or adoption, fostering or ovulation.

It happens. Hard things are hard.

She still carries around a bottle of oil, and, in my opinion,
too many phone chargers. She doesn't buy a pair of shoes
without texting me a picture first to ask if she will look old
in them. She swears up and down that I will be a mother one
day, and I suppose that I can indulge in her hope.

Hope is easier for her to carry than it is for me to believe it
for myself.

But I hope you're right, Mama.

*"You've got to get up every morning with a smile on your
face and show the world
All the love in your heart, then people gonna treat you better
You're gonna find, yes you will
That you're beautiful, as you feel."*

Carol King wrote the song *Beautiful* in 1971, and those
lyrics are what echoed from my mother's mouth into my
childhood bedroom most mornings. According to my very
reliable Google search, Carol wrote the song after observing
people on the New York City subway system. She

discovered her view of herself had a direct impact on how she treated other people. By treating other people with gratitude and respect, it allowed for her to feel beautiful in return.

Who could've known that a subway ride would turn into a song, or that a mother singing to her child would turn into an anthem of joy and a reminder to keep your head up, when all you want to do is hide in shame? My mother told me once that being a parent is unlike any joy she has ever known, and a heartache like no other, and a pride, and a sorrow, and it's all incredibly scary. She describes parenthood like a phantom pain. You know your child is out there, somewhere, but you can't always protect them, but when they sting with hurt, or failure, or embarrassment, or ache, you can feel it too.

13

A Table for Two

Somewhere on God's green earth, there is a picture of me
and my husband, posing seductively under the sparse shade
of a few pine trees. Kyle is leaned back against a tree with
one leg propped up, a la, the Marlboro Man, and I'm leaning
against him with my hand on his knee. With our heads titled
towards the sky and our eyes closed, I gave it my best,
damsel in distress, and we took our sexy Pinterest style
photo. This sounds great. It sounds like any other
engagement photo you would find on Instagram, but the
thing is…we are not those people. The steamy people who
stare into the camera with a smoldering passion and just
happened to be well dressed in a forest. *Nope.* It's not a
believable look on us. We looked like two stuffed sausage
dogs lying on top of each other. When the photographer
emailed them to us, I wet my pants laughing so hard and
promptly deleted it from my computer.

We are the kind of people who smile for photos as our
trusted dog, Stella, takes a dump in the background—that
actually happened, and that photograph is framed in our
bedroom. I tried to be disappointed that we aren't the sexy

posing kind, but I couldn't stop laughing long enough to care. When we took those photos, we had already been married for three years. We were having our pictures taken for Christmas cards, and we'd never had professional photos taken of us until that day.

When Kyle proposed to me, he sent me on a scavenger hunt in the middle of July. By the time I found him downtown, I was a sweaty mess, and my thunder thighs were so stuck with friction, they could've started a fire. I truly had no idea he was planning on asking me to marry him that day, not until I heard him call my name from across the street. When I turned around, I saw that he was wearing a sports coat and button-up shirt, but he was pale as a ghost in 96-degree heat. I didn't cry when we exchanged vows, but I couldn't stop blubbering when he popped the question on that hot July afternoon. I couldn't believe it. Someone who was so pure of heart, salt of the earth, and kind spirited, wanted to spend his days with me. To this day, I still don't understand what he sees in me, but I will be forever grateful that his hand fits like it was made to hold mine.

When our big day finally came, I stood in my childhood bedroom, and looked in the mirror as my mom began zipping up my wedding dress. I bought my dress online in a hurry, once I fully accepted the fact that I wasn't born with the bridal gene. On a Friday morning a few months earlier, I snuck off to *David's Bridal* to try on wedding dresses. I was alone and surrounded by women who were matching veils to trains, and I just didn't see the point. It wasn't for me. The dress was incredibly itchy and heavy. I just wanted a simple dress—an easy flow of fabric that I could wear a regular bra with and feel like myself in. I tried on my dress in our bathroom on a Saturday evening after FedEx delivered it, and I came very close to spilling a beer on the short train. It

was simple and white. All I needed really. I couldn't be
bothered with dresses or flowers; it was him I wanted. We
told very few friends and family of our plans, not wanting to
make a fuss and only wanting our parents as witnesses. I
wanted it to be a normal day, one that I would cherish as
long as I lived.

My mama zipped up my dress just as the lace snagged on a
loose piece of wood from an antique chest that sat at the foot
of my bed. She just knew that I was going to panic, but I
couldn't. I had a date to keep with my beloved. A friend
took simple photos of us and my mom's best friend became
ordained online to join us in holy matrimony. I'd ordered my
bouquet the day before and by a miracle they were able to
put together my order in such short notice. I hopped in the
car and drove around the lake I grew up on for the ten-
thousandth time and met him down by the water, in my
Pappaw's backyard.

He never took his eyes off of me, and I pray that I can
always remember every single detail of that day. We had a
small dinner with just our parents after we became man and
wife. And I think I kept waiting to hear an audible *snap* in
the air.

*Okay! I'm married now! Everything should feel perfect! I
should feel perfect! I should feel how everyone else looks!*

But it never usually works that way. Just because I married a
really good man didn't mean that we were always going to
have really good days. None of that is promised in vows.

From that day to now, not much has resembled a fairytale
like young newlyweds are led to believe. We've been poor
and not so poor, we've been let down and let go, we've been
sick and healthy, and we've been incredibly in love and

somedays, just in like. In sickness and in health, includes
mental health, but we didn't learn that until a few years in.
There has been silence and routine. Complacency and a type
of loneliness that we don't seem to mind. For a long while
after we were married, we didn't have a lot of friends or
confidence, so we just leaned on each other and the dreams
we had of better days ahead. Life comes at you fast, but the
pleasures of life that you reap, those take time.

I've learned to be patient when he is not. And vice versa. He
has learned to feed me even when I say I'm not hungry—
smart man. And we've both learned to lay down our
grudges, and that sometimes silence is better than getting
your way.

In our union, Kyle and I have had the same conversation
over and over, a conversation that not all couples are forced
to discuss. It had been three days since my first loss. I was
humiliated. I was broken. I was furious in a way that I
couldn't put words to. And he was...*fine*. He handled me
with kid gloves but was itching for me to be my old self
again. I stood in our kitchen and asked him if he was ever
going to show any emotion that matched mine. If he was
ever going to grieve. If he was ever going to give a damn
that his wife felt like a failure as a woman. If he was even
the tiniest bit of sad.

It was in that moment that he decided to share with me that
his mother had a few miscarriages when he was a kid. I'd
known he lost a baby sister; she was stillborn. I'd known he
was a miracle child. But I didn't know that he was so used to
pregnancy loss from his youth that this, "Was a drop in the
bucket."

I didn't kill him. I didn't claw out his eyes or rip out his
throat like I wanted. I did come very close to grabbing his
family jewels for a quick *pinch and twist*, but I refrained. I
just brought it to his attention that *I* had never been through
it at all. And he'd never been through it as the father of the
child. I can't remember how I exactly expressed this to him,
but I saw the lights come on in his eyes, and I knew he felt
terrible for the blundering of my emotions. We didn't speak
for a few days after that. I was too busy with slamming
doors and giving him the finger after he left the room. I had
to learn the hard way that men will never grieve the way
women do. They will never think the way women think.
They will never care the way women care. Not just about
pregnancy loss, but like…literally about anything. Men will
never be able to experience the emotional and physical pain
women feel. He has his own hurt, and his own way of
feeling that loss, but it will never be the same as mine.

We know what we know, now.

In my years of infertility, I've heard stories of men handling
their grieved wives or partners with clumsy hands after a
loss. Ladies, if this has happened to you, forgive those men.

They weren't built for the weight we carry.

Often times when we are out at restaurants, I look in the
corner of the hostess station to see if they have any
highchairs. Obviously, I don't need them for myself, but I've
just always wondered what it would be like to carry a
highchair to a table and pinch off small pieces of bread to
distract a child into contentment while adults dine. I've
watched couples, and families give babies their first lemons
as they pucker at the scratchy sourness, and everyone laughs.
I've also considered if parents ever truly get nervous or
embarrassed when their child throws a tantrum at the table

as other patrons try not to stare. After miscarriages, I always feel a little strange around kids or baby stuff. I started to feel like a creep in restaurants when I would stare at highchairs and the families who would request them. When you feel rejected by a plan that was squandered yet again, you do other things to fill your void and make yourself feel better. For us, that was sitting at the bar when we went out. You can do that when you don't have kids.

We could skip the wait for a corner booth and jump straight to the adult highchairs and watch baseball games and make small talk with the bartender. I told Kyle I liked sitting up there, and for a while that was the only place we would sit while we were out, and I would try to ignore the high-pitched squeals from toddlers on the other side of the room. There is something poetic about waiting at the bar for a table, we will upgrade when the time is right, one day, when there is a space available.

Marriage is weird. I met Kyle when I was twenty-two years old, and I didn't take him seriously at first. And now he is my family. He files our taxes and knows that I need my back cracked when I'm grumpy. He knows I'm only quiet when I'm nervous and I know that he will wake up in the night if his shoulders get cold. Without saying a word, I can tell when he is stressed. We both have never ending to-do lists, and getting his creepy varicose vein looked at is on the top of both of them. It is wild to me that ten years ago he was still a stranger, and now he can read my mind with just one look. He washed my hair for me when I couldn't find the energy to do it myself when depression suffocated our household, and he makes my coffee every Saturday morning.

When you exchange your vows, you have absolutely no idea what you're getting yourself into. I guess that's part of the excitement. My great-aunt Mavis was known for writing letters for big moments, and this is what she wrote to my grandparents, the day before they said *I do* in 1951.

Dear Faye & Bill,

This is the beginning of your future together. Now, you are one. May each day make you more and more happy. And as the sun sets each night, may you both be proud that you have each other.

I have never regretted one hour of married life and each year adds more to my happiness, and that is the reason I'm so sure that you both will find what I have.

To love, honor, and cherish, for the rest of your lives for so long as you both shall live is something to live up to and something to be proud of.

God has joined you two together and with Him helping you there should be success on every page of your lives. Just be thankful that God has given you both love. After all, that feeling you have deep down in your hearts for each other is to be cherished and just has to be given by someone out of this world. I wish you all the happiness in the world and you both are made of some mighty fine stuff. I hope to help you celebrate your golden wedding.

May the peace and happiness, and sorrows and joys, and troubles and care, and understanding and pleasures that make up each year of your lives together just bind you closer. Because as long as you have each other, you have

*everything. Live each day with every minute enjoyed for
each other.*

*Now, give each other a big kiss and it's happy sailing from
here on.*

Your big sister gives you her blessings,
Mavis Lou

Aunt Mavis nailed it once again. Well, I'm not so sure about
the happy sailing, but you see her point. There is peace,
happiness and joy, sorrows and troubles, heartache and
victory all found in a marriage. Honestly, that is all found in
the first month of marriage.

While we were cleaning out our office a few years ago, I
found an old box of cards that I'd saved over the years.
Glittered Christmas cards from my grandparents, birthday
cards I shamelessly shook to see if hidden money would fall
out, and anniversary cards filled the shoe box. I took the
time to read through them to decide which to keep a bit
longer and which ones I could toss. I picked up a blue card
with a globe on the front, not knowing what was inside. It
was a simple *thank you* card I'd written to Kyle. A short
thank you to him for taking such good care of me, and a
strong promise I swore to him was stamped at the bottom.

Kyle,

*I know I've been a handful lately, but I treasure you for the
way you take care of me. Thank you for sticking it out with
me. I love you.*

P.S. I promise you with all that I have, that one day, our
house will echo the laughter of children.

B

That promise seemed so easy to offer on the day I wrote that
card. Maybe I was on muscle relaxers, maybe my faith was
stronger than the days that followed, but I'm a woman of my
word. So, I will continue to do all that I can to give that
precious man children.

And until that day comes, until our number is called, we will
be waiting at the bar.

14

Here I Stand

It amazes me that I'm now so comfortable with the word *infertility*. I refused to say it for the longest time. Words like *infertility* and *miscarriage* feel harsh in my mouth. Those words roll around and struggle to cross my lips. The meaning of them just as bitter as they taste. Infertility is the loneliest thing that I've ever faced — a battle I've had to fight alone, a deserted path I've had to walk, never knowing where it would lead. It's hard to explain why or how I've felt so isolated, because I know that so many other women have faced this, too. I've met women who've experienced this heartache and even though we are armored up for the same war, they mirror the same feelings of confinement that match mine. As if we all received the same invitation but attended the party alone. How can we be so alone when there are so many?

A genetic specialist told me one time that I'm in the 1% of American women who have reoccurring, unexplained miscarriages. *One percent.* Unless you're a billionaire or an athletic protégé, you do not want to find yourself in a one percent margin. I'm no good with numbers. I've taken remedial math courses since the fourth grade, but there is no way that if *one in four* women have been affected by pregnancy loss, that it's just *one percent*. I stumbled through a rough explanation of that thought to the genetic specialist, and she said that I was on to something.

"Well, we've calculated the one-percent as the women who actually come forward and report multiple losses. Some women don't even tell their doctors they've had a loss at all, much less more than one."

The battle that rages as women fight for their health and families, is one that is fought mostly in silence. In my suffering I've laughed and cried, screamed at the top of my lungs and whispered prayers I didn't even think God could hear. My temper and demeanor have been just as lawless as my very person. I'm still standing. A little bent, never permanently broken, but I'm still here.

During all of my pregnancies, my husband would instantly start paying attention to my stomach. I overlooked my problem area and just let him talk to my bellybutton anyway. I was curious to see what he wanted to share with our bun. As he would leave for work my abdomen would receive a kiss before my lips. And after the dust settled from each loss, the going back to not touching my belly, or hearing Kyle tell them to have a good day, and to not make Mommy sick, was an added layer of loneliness I've never shared with anyone.

I thought by the time I finished this book my life may look a little different. I envisioned sending you off with joy, love and maybe, a pregnancy, fostering, or adoption announcement. Falling into the idea that you can't share your story until you know it has a happy ending.

But no. Not much here has changed. My spare room is still
empty and so are my arms. Our home has yet to echo the
sound of children laughing, but it's echoed many beautiful
sounds, still. Joy has filled moments, and moments have
sewn my days together in an extraordinary weave of beauty.
Now when people look at me through lenses of pity, I just
laugh.

Yes, this has been hard. And lonely. And embarrassing. And
on somedays, utterly hopeless. People still recommend
doggie-style sex positions to me, along with other odd
advice. Just last week someone introduced me to a woman
by saying, "Hey! She can't have kids either! Y'all should go
to dinner!"

But I've never felt more like myself. I'm painfully stretching
into the woman that I want to be, I trust my own voice, and
I've learned how and when to use it. I'm a full and complete
woman, even though I have no children. My days are just as
busy and fulfilling.

I still close my eyes sometimes and really try to picture it.
Motherhood.

I meditate on the day I might become a mother or what it
will feel like to hold a child's hand in mine. I imagine
chubby and sticky fingers covered in strawberry jam and
sweaty from a day spent at the park. I wonder if they will
have curly hair like me or if they will get my husband's deep
blue eyes. I've also dreamt of meeting a child my body
doesn't know. Wondering what it would be like to fall in
love with a child slowly over time as we get to know each
other. I lovingly hold all the daydreams and visions for
myself, and for all the women who dream of the same. I hold
my story in a firm grip. And I hold the faith that I've lost and

reclaimed inside a heart that's been broken and repaired time and time again.

My heart still leaps at the idea of being a mom—in the same way it leaps for a gorgeous sunset. In the same way it leaps for driving with the windows down on a fall morning, just like it does when my husband kisses me, or when I see the lake I grew up on, or when I embrace a friend for a good hug, or when I taste the first sip of wine after a long day. My heart leaps at the beauty of life. My heart has been broken, and so has my spirit, but I'm not done yet. You're not either.

Wherever you are, whatever you've lost—you're not done.

I breathe in a strong rhythm pretty regularly now. In fact, my favorite inhales are found when I'm alone on my back porch. I look up at the sweet gum tree that sways in the wind as I fill my lungs with that sweet Mississippi humidity. I exhale as I count my blessings, which are too many to name. I still have absolutely no idea why this is my journey, my story.

I may never know.

But I have to think it's because through all these losses, all the unknown, all the hurt—this was the way that I would find *me*.

I've learned to hold my shoulders back, with my tear-stained face, and cry out prayers through gritted teeth. I've learned that the women who have fought the same battle as me are tough as nails. I've learned that all is as it should be, even if it's hard. I've learned to listen to my gut, because she has never led me astray.

I'll stand here and hold my head as high as I can and know, that I'm just getting started.

And so are you.

Acknowledgments

I've been told that I'm a storyteller. I love a dramatic pause before delivering a good punchline. I love the anticipatory build before a pearl clutching shock. I've never shied away from telling a story, until the hardest story to tell, was my own. I can only assume the reason that I'm here, the reason I've faced the roads that I've walked, is because God knows exactly what He is doing, and He isn't known for making mistakes. No matter how hard the road gets, I will continue to tell stories as the ultimate Author unfolds them for me. In all my days, I will never be worthy of the love of Christ.

To my dear friend, Kellye Bolar, you're the first person to ever ask me when I was going to write my book. Until you had asked, I'd only held that idea as a dream and not a reality that I could actually pursue. Thank you for your friendship, your love and support, and for asking a question that encouraged me to do this. Lindsey Simmons, a beautiful friend who edited my words and told me to keep going when all I wanted to do was stop. I can't thank you enough for your invaluable friendship, and I will always be in awe of your obedience to our King. You are good people. You are my people. To Beth Morgan, for taking pictures of me and transforming them into images of a woman I can only hope I feel like one day. To Kristen Ley, for holding a torch for women and their success and fighting for them unlike anyone I know. To Kelsey Loftin, thank you for always answering my voice memos and for greeting my words with enthusiasm. Thank you for turning my inconsistent ramblings into beautiful designs. Thank you for taking on this project when you didn't have to. Thank you for telling me to do this. Thank you for feeding my enthusiasm of em dashes. You're treasured in my heart. To Catherine, Molly Gee, Germaine, & Meagan—my world somehow felt safer after our group got together. I thank each of you for your support, humor, love, and examples of how to grip life by the horns and demand what you want from her. I'm grateful for each of you. To Sarah, Haley Jo, Kathryn, Christina, Taylor, Hardy, Nikki, Kristina, Ashley, JoBeth, & Haley— you each add such a value to my life that is indispensable. I prayed for good friends for a long time, and each of you are the answers to such prayers. To Lauren Bird, for loving me from across the world, for matching my pain, for hearing me out. You're a treasure I hope to meet one day. To my sisters, Leslie and Albree—thank you for showing me what strength in the face of heartache looks like. May the Lord bless and keep you.

To Ashley, David, Jonathan, Denise, Debra, Tim, and Keith—some of the best stories I have hold each of you in them. I've no idea what we did to deserve each other in this life, or how we scored such awesome parents and grandparents, but I'm eternally grateful that y'all are my kin.

To my parents, Rick and Diane, you are my people, my home base, and my favorite necks to hug. The root of my being is found in the pleasure of being your child, and I will forever be thankful that I get the honor of calling you Mom & Dad. We are far from perfect, but I would choose both of you, time and time again, and twice on Sunday.

To my husband, Henry, you are the best part of me. I can never thank you enough for encouraging me through this process. Thank you for listening to me read aloud the same paragraph for forty-five minutes until it sounded right. Thank you for never complaining about the glow of my computer screen in the middle of the night. Thank you for holding my hand through every loss. Thank you for charging my phone after I've fallen asleep. Thank you for believing that we will be parents one day. Thank you for giving me permission to break bowls, so I don't break myself. Thank you for loving me. Thank you for all of it. I'm madly in love with a really good man, and in case I forget to tell you later, I had a really good time.

For Bill and Faye Massey, I hope I made you proud.